Is fatigue your middle name? Are you running on empty?
Are you determined to go from a tired observer
to a vibrant participant in your own life?

If you've picked up this book, your answer is likely a resounding
YES! This comprehensive guide enables fibromyalgia patients to
help reverse chronic fatigue by recognizing its myriad manifestations...

- Do you suffer from overwhelming fatigue...even when you're already lying down?

- Are you exhausted by the simplest daytime activities?

- Do you wake up frequently during the night?

- Do you suffer from panic attacks or a feeling of impending doom?

- Do you have a drug-like craving for food?

- Is your skin cool, clammy, and prone to sweating?

- Do you feel disconnected from your body, as if you're in a dream?

- Are you hypersensitive to lights, sounds, or odors?

- Do your legs feel heavy, as if you are carrying a heavy load?

- Are you in a constant brain fog with difficulty concentrating and remembering?

∽

If you are all too familiar with these symptoms,
it's time to find out...

WHAT YOUR DOCTOR MAY *NOT* TELL YOU ABOUT FIBROMYALGIA FATIGUE

Please turn this page for praise for Dr. St. Amand's
What Your Doctor May *Not* Tell You About Fibromyalgia...

"I have seen the magic of guaifenesin and the program in WHAT YOUR DOCTOR MAY *NOT* TELL YOU ABOUT FIBROMYALGIA work."
—Devin Starlanyl, author of *The Fibromyalgia Advocate*

"Dr. St. Amand's unique approach to fibromyalgia gives patients who have run out of treatment options a new hope. . . . A revelation to fibromyalgics."
—Miryam Erlich Williamson, author of *Fibromyalgia: A Comprehensive Approach* and *The Fibromyalgia Relief Book*

"Offers a clear road map out of the wilderness of fibromyalgia pain and fatigue."
—Kendall Gerdes, M.D., former president, American Academy of Environmental Medicine

"I've been using guaifenesin and the protocol in this book in my practice for seven years. The results have been amazing! If you have fibromyalgia I strongly recommend you buy this book and begin treatment immediately."
—C. Ronald McBride, M.D., assistant clinical professor of medicine, UCLA Medical Group

"Groundbreaking...Dr. St. Amand's research will permit fibromyalgia to become merely a memory."
—Dr. John Willems, M.D., head, Division of Obstetrics and Gynecology, Scripps Clinic

WHAT YOUR DOCTOR MAY *NOT* TELL YOU ABOUT™

FIBROMYALGIA FATIGUE

The Powerful Program That
Helps You Boost Your Energy
and Reclaim Your Life

R. PAUL ST. AMAND, M.D.
and CLAUDIA CRAIG MAREK

WARNER BOOKS

An AOL Time Warner Company

The information in this book is not intended to be a substitute for individual medical diagnosis and advice, and should not be followed without first consulting a health care professional. You are advised to consult with your physician regarding matters relating to your health, particularly if you have any special conditions requiring attention, before implementing this or any other program or therapy.

Copyright © 2003 by The St. Amand Trust and Claudia Craig Marek, M.A.
All rights reserved.

Warner Books, Inc., 1271 Avenue of the Americas, New York, NY 10020
Visit our Web site at www.twbookmark.com

W An AOL Time Warner Company

Printed in the United States of America

First Printing: October 2003
10 9 8 7 6 5 4 3 2 1

Library of Congress Cataloging-in-Publication Data
St. Amand, R. Paul.
    What your doctor may not tell you about fibromyalgia fatigue : the powerful program that helps you boost your energy and reclaim your life / R. Paul St. Amand and Claudia Craig Marek.
        p. cm.
    Includes index.
    ISBN 0-446-67730-2
    1. Chronic fatigue syndrome. 2. Fibromyalgia—Complications. I. Marek, Claudia. II. Title.

RB150.F37S72 2003
616.7'4—dc21   2003045045

Book design by Charles A. Sutherland
Cover design by Diane Luger

Contents

———————— ◈ ————————

Preface

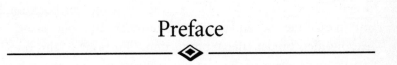

For many years there were several doctors in my life. Some cared that my body was full of pain and that many of my symptoms did not respond to the prescribed treatments; others felt that I was overreacting, and they referred me to two psychiatrists and one psychologist. They were helpful in some ways but unable to decide that my illness was mental. The psychologist, a woman, was the most helpful. She acknowledged my problems and said that I had a high tolerance for pain and was a strong person although my search for the right doctor was not finished. After sixteen years of actively seeking help my condition continued to deteriorate. By 1991 my body was bedridden for 50 percent of the time, and for 10 percent of the time I felt reasonable, and the other 40 percent of the time I dragged myself around. Guilt is deep in ourselves when we battle this mind-draining disease.

—*Lora V., Arizona*

Tired? We know you are. This is why we wrote this book for you: to examine and explain how fibromyalgia and other associated disorders hinder energy production. Our primary aim is to raise your awareness of their interweaving assaults on your body. The obstacles we list are separate conditions, but each adversely impacts your already depleted energy. While the reversal of fibromyalgia may take time, there's no reason to delay working on other conditions that can be remedied. Thus our immediate goal is to improve your resilience in daily coping while urging you to work toward long-term correction of *all* deficits. Be aware that there's often no quick fix. Though all may be genetic propensities, they're certainly helped along by failing to take them seriously at their onset, the very time when correction is easiest.

If you've already been diagnosed with fibromyalgia, you know that the majority of doctors and health-care providers will tell you that you need to "get over it" or "learn to live with it," since there's "nothing that can be done." To this we thumb our noses (in lieu of some basic profanities—all of which we've heard in the course of our practice). This simply isn't true, and it's likely the cause for the high ongoing rate of depression in people with fibromyalgia, even after their illness has begun its reversal. So why do well-meaning physicians so often steer their patients in the wrong direction? It's certainly not out of malice or any agenda the doctor has. Most physicians truly want to see their patients healthy and happy. It's simply that they don't understand myriad layers of fibromyalgia.

The medical industry has come a long way in understanding how fibromyalgia works—even in the years since our first book, *What Your Doctor May* Not *Tell You About Fibromyalgia,* was published in late 1999. Even our practice has had to reexamine and rethink its treatment protocol. At first we were so pleased with reversing so many of the symptoms of this challenging illness that we ourselves didn't address the energy issue fully. Time, patients' insistence, and a clearer understanding of this devastating component have helped us better accept the simple fact that no fibromyalgic should suffer from energy deprivation.

None of us needs to be told that illnesses induce fatigue. We expect physical stresses such as the common cold, flu, allergies, surgeries, or prolonged mental stress to steal our energy. Our bodies can produce only so much, and anything that requires us to use more than we can manufacture will eventually deplete our reserves.

The way we protect our reserves is by avoiding expenditures that arise regularly from disease, stress, poor nutrition, and excesses such as alcohol, drugs, smoking, and other bad habits. Healthy people find it relatively easy to hoard adequate energy surpluses. Avoiding overwhelming demands on reserves lets the body waltz through unexpected emotional upsets, illnesses, or injuries. Simply put, energy stores are somewhat like checking accounts in that we make deposits and withdrawals. In our metabolic economy, positive balances are necessary, and we can safeguard supplies only by limiting consumption.

Our maximal energy potential is genetically determined: Each of us operates within individual and finite limits. That's the way it is for all animal life, and humans are no exception. We all know people who have great excesses of energy and others who have lamentably less capacity than our own. The sole purpose of this book is to help you draw from your own, best, sources of energy, without suffering from debilitating deprivation.

Any illness is inopportune, but most are either self-healing or at least treatable with help from capable professionals. Horrible injuries and even major illnesses eventually heal to some degree. Unfortunately, people with fibromyalgia suffer almost continuous energy failure. Even relatively minor mental or physical stresses can cause them to collapse—being, in effect, the proverbial straw that breaks the camel's back.

Because fibromyalgia is so overwhelming, we're often oblivious to the initially imperceptible warning signals being whispered by the likes of diabetes and hypoglycemia. They seem innocuous in their early phases. Obesity and lipid problems are other conditions that may well reflect our lifelong indulgences as much as our genetic propensities, but certainly with a little knowledge they can be conquered and controlled.

Unlike our first book, *What Your Doctor May* Not *Tell You About Fibromyalgia,* in which we discuss the disease in detail and outline a program for reversing it, in this book we will not go into quite as much detail regarding the disease. We refer you back to that original text for more sweeping theories and specifics about beginning reversal. We suggest you use this newer book as a supplement. It should help you boost your energy levels and to make positive changes in your health.

To make this concept easier for you to follow, we'll be using the metaphor of a well-balanced bicycle wheel. There are many much, much smaller wheels in every cell of your body. They were designed and quality structured to withstand most stresses we encounter. Each condition we'll discuss can potentially damage at least one spoke of those internal, energy-producing rotators. Altering one such spoke won't totally stop the wheel from functioning, but it will place a heavier burden upon the remaining support rods. Weaken or destroy a second or third spoke and the working ones will certainly get unduly burdened. The resulting stress eventually causes wobble and, ultimately, system breakdown.

Because fibromyalgics often find their situation compounded by other conditions, such as hypoglycemia, weight problems, diabetes, hormone fluxes, high cholesterol, and other ancillary conditions, this book will also address these conditions and the toll they take on energy production. Like the bicycle wheel, all systems must be in balance for the body's energy production to "perfectly cycle."

Most of you reading these pages are already well aware of your energy shortages. You may have been accurately diagnosed with fibromyalgia. What may have escaped your attention, and the attention of your health professional, is the link between this and other conditions just mentioned. Much like credit card debt with added interest charges and penalties, these illnesses, when combined, rapidly deplete our energy savings accounts. The eventual collapse is a bit like the sequential fall of successive dominoes.

Many of you will struggle with some of the concepts we're going to describe. They're not always easy to comprehend, but we've done our best to simplify them. This book will outline the most common health barriers that fibromyalgics tend to face when trying to boost their energy. You may find it helpful to discuss this book with your doctor or medical practitioner, so that you may work together to improve your overall health.

Over the years, we've learned most of what we know from people like you—our patients. We dedicate this book mainly to them, but also to newcomers who've just filed for metabolic bankruptcy. Our approach is designed as a chance to reorganize your depleted energy finances and even reestablish your good credit rating. We'll help you learn what changes *you* can make to overcome your current energy deficits. As you'll see, reinforcing even one spoke on the wheel will help. So why not stay with us, and take a shot at reclaiming your energy?

—R. Paul St. Amand, M.D.
—Claudia Craig Marek
Marina del Rey, California

Acknowledgments

———————◆———————

We would like to acknowledge several people without whom this book would not have been possible. First of course, we owe our families a debt of gratitude for the time we've stolen for this project. Once again, Mari Florence's expertise was pivotal in bringing this book to fruition. Diana Baroni, our tireless and talented editor, and Carol Mann, our always gentle and supportive agent, also deserve our heartfelt thanks.

Gloria Martinez and Malcolm Potter provided invaluable assistance, in our office, tabulating statistics, and with this manuscript.

Our patients and all those who have thoughtfully confided in us added greatly to our finished product, and our gratitude extends to them, each and every one.

Claudia Gray and Lou Marek used their artistic talents to produce some of our illustrations. We also thank them for their contributions.

WHAT YOUR DOCTOR
MAY *NOT* TELL YOU
ABOUT™
FIBROMYALGIA
FATIGUE

◆

First Things First:
The Fibromyalgia Reversal Protocol

Before addressing specific energy-related issues, it's important to confirm that you have fibromyalgia. Such a diagnosis should come from a health-care professional who is familiar with the illness. Your physician, chiropractor, physiotherapist, or physician's assistant may be quite competent at spotting it. Once you get verification, we urge you to launch into the protocol we outlined in our first book, *What Your Doctor May* Not *Tell You About Fibromyalgia.*

Everything you're going to read in this book can be implemented while you are using the protocol outlined in our first book. This book is designed to help you combat energy deficiencies from fibromyalgia, which are increasingly the most common complaints we hear. We'll also cover some of the other energy drains that often sneak in as by-products of related disorders. If you choose to skip the sections about our protocol for reversing fibromyalgia, you'll still find the rest of the information in this book insightful. However, it's fair to warn you that *partial* compliance may provide only temporary

Band-Aids and subpar resolution of your symptoms. We've found that the long-term way back to feeling your best is to get with the total program.

If you already own a copy of *What Your Doctor May Not Tell You About Fibromyalgia,* we urge you to become totally familiar with chapter 6. This current book is intended as a useful companion to complete the search for your defaulted energy. The original book does, however, contain more details concerning the illness. We won't repeat it all here, though we will summarize the main points as a recap for people familiar with fibromyalgia and also as an introduction for those unfamiliar with our protocol.

Dragging through life isn't much fun, as you've already found out. The following overview should get you started reversing your fibromyalgia. It's an outline of the steps you must take to begin its correction.

FIND A DOCTOR WHO CAN MAKE THE DIAGNOSIS

I have had the symptoms of fibro since the birth of my second child nine years ago. I had a physician who did not believe fibro exists, let alone try to treat it. He had me believing I was going crazy!! Finally, after just getting worse I found a new family doctor that was willing to take me on. She was *very* knowledgeable about fibro and had read the guai protocol. She encouraged me to give it a try when I told her I had read your book. I have been on it eleven months and can't believe the change in my life. . . . I have energy and most of my symptoms are gone. My doctor encouraged me to keep a journal of my progress. I read it the other day and I am amazed at how far I have come. As one of your patients commented in the book, "Just take it and go on with your life and it will work." They were not kidding.

—*Kathy H., New Brunswick, Canada*

As we said in the beginning, you've got to be sure you're suffering from fibromyalgia. This seems obvious, even silly, but it is important. Lots of other conditions have similar complaints. It's also dangerous to treat yourself and to assume that all your symptoms are from this single entity. If you haven't been diagnosed, call and make an appointment with your primary doctor after reading this chapter. When you phone, make sure to mention you suspect you have fibromyalgia. If the staff suggests that the doctor doesn't believe such a thing exists or is reluctant to treat it, don't make the appointment. Call a different physician. This may seem harsh, but you'll need a sympathetic doctor who will work with you. The road to recovery can be difficult, and you'll need a good driver. You can't expect that a closed mind can properly read the directions needed to guide you to your destination.

If you need help finding a doctor, there are several things you can try. First of all, ask your friends. If one of them identifies a physician who's particularly open-minded and a good listener, start there. Luckily, you don't have to have a highly limited specialist to make the diagnosis of fibromyalgia. Family doctors and other primary-care practitioners, including chiropractors, are perfectly qualified to do it. Precisely because they aren't narrowly specialized, general practitioners may have acquired fewer preconceived notions.

Another possibility for finding a doctor is to call a local fibromyalgia support group. If there are no FM groups in your area, try the local chapter of The Arthritis Foundation. It usually keeps lists of doctors who are understanding and sympathetic to fibromyalgics. Your local hospital medical staff office may be aware of an interested practitioner. You can also sift through on-line newsgroups or Web sites for good leads. Any physician or nurse practitioner licensed in your particular state can help administer the medication we will describe, guaifenesin (gwī fen é sin).

Before your initial appointment, compile your symptoms from lists in this book. Keep it simple and avoid dramatic details. Be sure to provide your doctor the names of all of your current medications and supplements. Reveal all over-the-counter preparations you use—for example, analgesics such as aspirin, acetaminophen, and nonsteroidal anti-inflammatory drugs (NSAID) that include Advil, Aleve, ibuprofen, and so on. In particular, don't hold back telling about herbal supplements such as St.-John's-wort, echinacea, and *Ginkgo biloba.* If you're taking more unusual products such as Heal-all or Energy Boost, it's important to write down what they contain. Be honest about the amounts you take. Your new physician will need to know exactly what you're using, especially if you're going to be given new prescriptions for anything.

It isn't a wise move to try to cram our protocol down some poor doctor's throat on the first visit. Your doctor will need to take into account your particular medical history and condition. Our information may be entirely new to him or her. You've been boning up on the subject and might well be better prepared than the physician. Be mindful of your top priority, which is finding a supportive doctor to help you. If your introductory approach is gentle enough, you've got a better chance of working together in the future. Especially avoid acting like the chief instructor who's trying to take immediate charge of the encounter. Use the same sweet ways you'd use when trying to establish a relationship with, say, a new date. Doctors are patsies for charm and warmth just like anybody else.

Down the line, you certainly have the mission of helping to teach your physician. It's fine to provide doctors with reading material, but immediately thrusting a whole book at them is a little intimidating. It suggests that you're very demanding and that your particular needs take priority over everything else they have to read and do. After a visit or two, it's okay to refer to whatever we've printed that pertains to you. Use subsequent visits to gradually interject what facts you've learned by reading. It's also the time to offer the observations that you'll make during the course of your treatment. However, the very best method of convincing a professional is by getting better while you're under medical supervision. Results are great teachers. Just get well and watch how quickly your doctor responds. Other fibromyalgics under his or her care will greatly profit by your diligence and diplomacy!

Once you're face to face with your chosen doctor, what should you expect? The diagnosis of fibromyalgia is properly made in three parts. It begins by taking a detailed medical history and reviewing all your body's systems. Since fibromyalgia causes such diverse complaints as fatigue, depression, irritable bowel syndrome, irritable bladder, numbness, leg cramps, headaches, palpitations, and more, the doctor will want to ask you about these and other symptoms, as well. Many doctors use check sheets that allow them to sequentially screen for a host of symptoms. Try to establish a rough chronology of when your problems first appeared and a time frame that will suggest the rate of progression of your illness. This time line will also serve to monitor your improvement once you begin reversing the illness with the medication we suggest using, guaifenesin.

When your doctor is satisfied that your symptoms and history suggest fibromyalgia, the second step will be to examine you with that diagnosis in mind. Though many doctors may not feel comfortable using our "mapping" technique, they should at least do a hands-on examination looking for the so-called tender points. This search is especially revealing for both patient and examiner if either of them thinks they're dealing with the so-called chronic fatigue syndrome and not fibromyalgia. Tenderness depends too much on individual pain thresholds, and we therefore much prefer a thorough body search for the distinctive muscular findings that exist in fibromyalgia. We'll describe those shortly. But whichever course your doctor chooses, be aware that you must be physically examined to confirm the diagnosis.

If you haven't had basic blood work recently, it will probably be ordered as the final step in making the diagnosis. Because there are no blood tests for fibromyalgia, these are ordered only to ensure that nothing else is causing your symptoms, and therefore will vary from patient to patient, and physician to physician. Testing usually includes blood counts to rule out anemia or infection, and a thyroid test known as TSH, for checking thyroid function. An underactive thyroid can cause many symptoms, including extreme fatigue. A fasting blood sugar will look for diabetes. This condition can cause rapid swings in blood glucose, enough to produce many symptoms. Other tests will rule out liver disease, kidney problems, various forms of arthritis, and lupus. High calcium levels can cause muscle pain, and a high uric acid would denote gout. Your physician won't want to jump to conclusions without eliminating other conditions that cause fatigue or muscular aching.

If you're a woman above the age of fifty, your doctor may want to do a sedimentation ("sed") rate. This blood test screens for many kinds of inflammation and is the only test that will detect polymyalgia rheumatica, an unrelated condition with symptoms quite similar to those of fibromyalgia. This test is especially important, because failure to expeditiously diagnose and aggressively treat polymyalgia can result in blindness or stroke. The treatment for this condition is *not* the same as for fibromyalgia.

Finally, armed with a review of your past history, current symptoms, physical examination, and test results, both you and your doctor should feel more secure with the diagnosis of fibromyalgia. So now it's time for the first step, which is to document your starting point before you embark on our protocol to treat and reverse your illness.

MAP YOUR LUMPS AND BUMPS

I found my first body map to be a powerful experience. As I looked at the marks on the paper I felt a sudden sense of vindication—for the first time I could see something concrete, see proof that something real was causing my pain. After so many hundreds of tests coming back normal, this was a relief. The realization hit me that someone else believed that my pain could be real, that it wasn't coming from some overly dramatic nervous system, or too-sensitive nerve fibers, or any of the other crazy theories I'd heard espoused over the years.

—*Susie, Los Angeles, California*

We've introduced a system of physical examination in our previous books that we call mapping. It may well be foreign to your doctor or your other body therapists. If you can find someone who will learn or who is already skilled in the technique, you're way ahead. It makes it far easier to identify your guaifenesin dosage requirements and to confirm your steady reversal. Without mapping, all you will have to go on are the hours or days of improvement that eventually appear. Using our method to feel clearing areas won't leave you so totally on your own trying to interpret your progress. Especially during tougher reversing days, only a map can verify that you're moving favorably ahead. Thus, if you can find someone to map you, you'll have two sets of clues: your surges of feeling better and the objective findings in tissue lumps and bumps as they're breaking up.

If you want to be mapped, and your physician does not feel sufficiently skilled to do it, there are alternatives. Ask your doctor to help you find someone he or she trusts, a professional with "good hands" such as a chiropractor, or a physical or massage therapist. You should certainly select a person who has worked on fibromyalgics or is quick to learn. This team approach is usually very effective. The mapping person will monitor your physical progress while your doctor observes the facets of fibromyalgia that can't be felt with hands. Such combined professional efforts make it easier to meticulously adjust the dosage of medication.

In the unlikely event that your doctor has no suggestions,

ask your friends for a referral to someone they know. Local support groups are usually extremely helpful in directing your search—they're quite aware of people who have the required skills. Don't hesitate to ask about experience when you make your appointment. It's often easier to find someone who will map than to locate an open-minded physician willing to work with guaifenesin. We strongly suggest that you don't skip this step.

When you go to your first mapping appointment, you should bring a copy of the "before treatment" illustration we provide in this chapter. The caricature displays the sites usually involved and helps direct the examiner's manual search for your personal distribution. The first map is very important, and ideally made before you begin testing guaifenesin. If you're already taking the medication, mapping can still be done frequently during your treatment. Each subsequent examination will serve as comparison with the previous ones. Especially in the early days of reversal, this process is the only sure way to determine improvement.

Body workers such as those listed above are all accustomed to palpating muscles, ligaments, and tendons. They know abnormal tissue when they feel it and should be able to draw something representing their findings on the body map. We draw the lesions as we feel them beginning in the upper body and working toward the feet. We sketch our findings according to location and size; by pressing harder with our pen, we darken the area more heavily when we want to illustrate harder spots. It's not mandatory for your examiner to use our system. He or she may have a personal method that will serve quite adequately for future comparisons. It's imperative, however, that the mapping include only abnormalities objectively felt by the

PATIENT: _____ DATE: _____

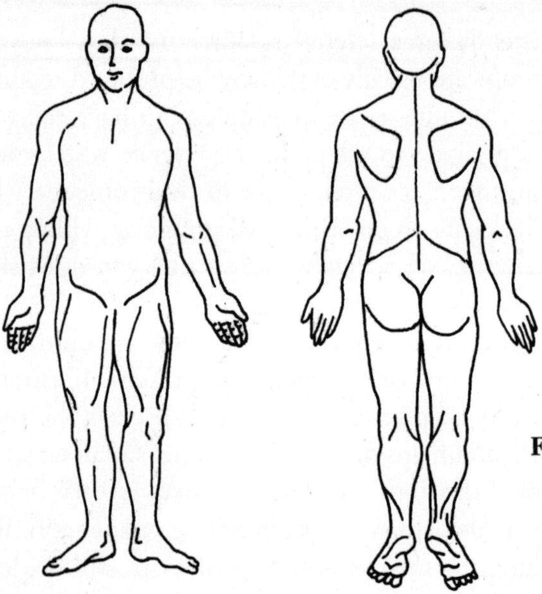

Figure 1

___ Fatigue
___ Irritability
___ Nervousness
___ Depression
___ Insomnia
___ Impaired
  Concentration
___ Impaired Memory
___ Anxiety
___ Salt Craving
___ Sweating
___ Gas
___ Palpitations
___ Frontal
  Headaches
___ Occipital
  Headaches
___ General
  Headaches

___ Dizziness
  ___ a) Vertigo
  ___ b) Imbalance
  ___ c) Faintness
___ Blurred Vision
___ Eye Irritation
___ Nasal
  Congestion
___ Abnormal Tastes
  ___ a) Bad
  ___ b) Metallic
___ Ringing Ears/
  Tinnitus
___ Numbness
___ Restless Legs
___ Leg Cramps
___ Nausea
___ Bloating
___ Constipation

___ Diarrhea
___ Dysuria
___ Pungent Urine
___ Bladder
  Infections
___ Vulvodynia
___ Weight Gain
___ Brittle Nails
___ Bruising
___ Itching
___ Rashes
___ Sensitivities
  ___ a) Chemical
  ___ b) Light
  ___ c) Odor
  ___ d) Sounds
  ___ e) Allergies
___ Growing Pains
___ Pain

The last step before you begin taking the med
guaifenesin is extremely important. A thorou
licylates in all your medications, supplemen
skin products (topicals) is absolutely nec

In order for guaifenesin to work,
access to receptors in the kidneys
products we use every day, such
tritional and herbal supplem
are chemicals known as s
fenesin's access to the
blocked, none of the
Thus salicylates
this step. The
point in eve

The b
thing
icati

guaifenesin
very reluctantly gave up my barley green and pycn̶o̶g̶
but felt not much different after I had done this. Don't
even ask about the skin and hair products I exchanged.
Now I have a group of about thirty people, and through
our consistent self-effort and determination we are all
getting well! We are not just enduring and hanging in
with gritted teeth. We're reclaiming our health and actively living our lives as a celebration rather than an obstacle course.

—*Miki K., Kauai, Hawaii*

...ication called
...gh search for sa-
...ts, and beauty and
...essary.

...t must have unrestricted
... Many ingredients in the
...as lipsticks, muscle balms, nu-
...ents, cosmetics, and sunscreens
...licylates. These totally block guai-
...renal receptors. When this access is
...drugs we use is of any benefit whatsoever.
...ust be carefully avoided. You cannot ignore
...e are no shortcuts, and without it there is no
...n beginning guaifenesin.

...est way to check your products is to gather up every-
...n the house that you use on your body or take as a med-
...on or supplement. You'll undoubtedly clear out most of
...ur bathroom's contents, so make time when you won't be
disturbed. You'll need to use this book and a regular dictionary
or a book on cosmetic ingredients, because you're going to
learn to read the labels on all products you use. You'll probably also need a magnifying glass, because the print on some
packaging is impossibly small. Sometimes only active ingredients are listed; in this case, you must contact the manufacturer
for the names of all the *inactive* components. (See the back of
this book for a list of common natural salicylates as of our writing of this book.)

- Go through all your medications. For prescription and
  over the counter drugs check the chemical names. For example, Tylenol (acetaminophen) is okay, Pepto Bismol

(bismuth subsalicylate) is a blocker. You do not need to check inactive ingredients such as cellulose or food color.

- Check topical creams for salicylate, or plant extracts such as aloe, camphor, or menthol. Many items such as topical analgesics, wart removers, dandruff shampoos, and skin treatments harbor salicylate by name.
- Though vitamins and minerals are safe they should be scrutinized for herbal additives such as St.-John's-wort, ginseng, rosemary, parsley, and more.
- Don't assume that an herb or mint flavoring hasn't been added to a hormone such as DHEA or melatonin.
- Pharmacists as well as on-line pharmacology and other reputable Web sites can help you greatly.
- Check every product in your bathroom. Mouthwashes, toothpastes, soaps, shampoos, conditioners, razors, shaving creams, deodorants, nasal sprays, lotions, toners, tanning agents, masks, ointments, suppositories, acne medications, and so forth all need to be scrutinized. Check all dental hygiene, breath freshener, and gum-care products for natural or artificial mint flavoring, or plant oils such as clove. Lip balms and sunscreens often contain salicylates by name or as the newer term, *octisalate.* Others may have included aloe or castor oil to satisfy the current natural-is-good craze.
- All plants make salicylates—that's how they get out of the ground alive. You can't afford to have them bleed on you, however, because salicylate *will* enter your body through intact skin. Buy hard rubber or canvas gloves to avoid contact with plant oils and saps while doing heavy gardening. If you dislike working with heavy gloves, try the thin latex variety used by doctors and readily found in pharmacies.

Keep them handy so that you won't feel too lazy to look for them and get tempted to work barehanded.

You'll end up with three piles of products: those you can use, those you must discard, and a third questionable group that doesn't list ingredients. If you feel married to any of the latter group, you'll have to call manufacturers for information, or contact them via their Web sites. Use no product if you don't safely recognize all of its contents. If it's something you'll suck on, don't buy it unless the manufacturer reveals whether or not mint or menthol has been added. Remember that both synthetic and natural mint are salicylates.

BEGIN TAKING GUAIFENESIN

There is a moral here for us, I think. If I hadn't asked for the guai, none of it would have been initiated by him. I think physicians are out there who care about healing their patients and who may know that conventional medicine doesn't do all it can. If we don't initiate these discussions (and be prepared to be shot down by the closed-minded ones out there), we may never get these doctors to be comfortable prescribing these treatments. We as patients can help them along their way to feeling comfortable with other treatments. Of course, it takes an open-minded physician. I know I am fortunate to have found this doctor.

—*Beth, Florida*

Throughout the years that we have been researching and treating fibromyalgia, we have used several different drugs, with varied results. In 1992, our search led us to guaifenesin, a widely available medication. We have used guaifenesin to develop a treatment protocol that addresses the actual disturbance caused by our defective genes, and not merely its symptoms. We have treated thousands of patients successfully with this medication. If your physician doesn't seem to know much about this medication, be sure to mention that it has no significant side effects when taken properly. He or she can always look it up in the *Physician's Desk Reference* for more specific, technical information, or turn to our Web site for more complete information (www.fibromyalgiatreatment.com).

Until 2002, guaifenesin was available mostly by prescription, with some weaker strengths for sale over the counter. However, that all changed when, in July 2002, the FDA lifted the restrictions because guaifenesin was known to be extremely safe. As a result, at the time of this writing, both 600 and 1200 mg. strengths are on the market as over the counter medications. A patent for these "new" guaifenesins was granted to one company, Adams, and named "Mucinex." Mucinex is a long-acting guaifenesin and should be taken in two daily doses, approximately twelve hours apart. Despite what pharmacy labels may say, in our experience we have found that breaking or cutting the tablet in half for precise dosing doesn't compromise the benefits we anticipate. If you decide to use the lower strengths, which come in capsule or tablet form, they are short-acting preparations and should be taken three times a day instead.

It is inevitable, we hope, that other brands of guaifenesin will come on the market as time passes, but they will also be over the counter due to the FDA ruling. This is both good news and bad news. The good news is that a doctor's prescription is no longer required, but it also means that insurance coverage is no longer available to cover the costs. In the resource section in the back of the book you'll find some places to get guaifenesin at the best possible prices.

Finding Your Dosage

It's important to be systematic in establishing your dosage. We can't emphasize this enough. When it comes to your health, why create a guessing game? If you're not methodical in establishing your own requirements, some glaring uncertainties face you. You may get advice from other patients or support-group members to either raise or lower your dose based on how you feel on a given day. *But don't just disregard your doctor's advice.* You wouldn't do it with your blood pressure medicine, so don't do it with your guaifenesin. Not to mention the fact that *it's generally unwise to change dosages of any medication without sanction from your doctor.* Otherwise you often end up with two very confused people: you and your physician.

In the early weeks of treatment, it's a good idea to keep track of what's going on by writing information on a small calendar. To make it easier to track good- and bad-day patterns, make a few daily notations, and keep them simple. Possible entries might read: "headache ½ day," "more energy in the A.M.," "back better," "shoulder stopped hurting," or "neck very sore." It's tempting to rate days on a scale of one to ten for each and every symptom, especially pain. This may seem like a good system in the beginning. Eventually, however, you'll realize that the ratings' significance becomes blurred. After runs of several good weeks, it's difficult to remember and compare the intensity of current and past cycles. Down the line, your worst day may be considerably better than your best day before starting treatment.

Start by taking 300 mg. of guaifenesin twice a day. This will require cutting or breaking your 600 mg. tablets in half. From our experience, it's extremely rare that less will work as effectively. We have seen only a very few patients reverse with lower amounts. If you're concerned with being "very sensitive to medications," 300 mg. twice a day is already a low dosage for guaifenesin, one quarter of the FDA approved amount.

Hold at 300 mg. twice a day for the *first week*. If you get distinctly worse, you may already have found the yellow-brick road to recovery. Let's stress this from the beginning: *When you reach your required dosage, your symptoms will get worse.* Worse is good! For example, if you're tired, you may become exhausted. If you ache, you'll hurt even more. Symptoms that were mild or barely noticeable before may now bother you more intensely. This happens because reversal time is so much faster than the time it took to develop fibromyalgia. It's an accelerated process that for the same reason may produce aches and pains from sites you never felt before. Past cycles may have been gentler ones that operated somewhat below your perception in certain areas. We've each been given a pain threshold; you likely must exceed your own before you feel pain.

If you don't feel distinctly worse during the first week at 300 mg. twice a day, you should double your dosage to a full 600 mg. tablet twice a day, a total of 1200 mg. a day. We generally instruct our patients to do this automatically if they can't feel a distinct difference during the first, low-dosage week. You'll usually notice the expected exacerbation of symptoms within three to fourteen days once the medication is tailored for you. At 1200 mg. a day, 70 percent of our patients start feeling the exacerbation of their symptoms that signals they've started their reversal.

We utilize the advantage that mapping provides once our patients have been on guaifenesin for one month or so. If you or your examiner notices no appreciable difference after that time, increase to 1800 mg. a day. This amount of medication usually proves sufficient to initiate reversal in 90 percent of our patients. As we stated, feeling worse during treatment is an expected result from having successfully found your proper dosage.

If you've been at 1800 mg. a day for another month and nothing has changed—neither worse nor better days—and this is confirmed by a repeat mapping, you should again discuss with your doctor whether to raise your dosage, this time to 1200 mg. twice a day. In our experience, this will take care of more than 95 percent of patients. Just as before, hold this dose for another month. If there is no change in your condition, you may be one of the rare people who require even higher amounts, 3600 or even 4800 mg. per day.

Because success is so high at 1800 and especially 2400 mg., lack of change for better or worse is strongly suggestive of blocking by absorbing some source of salicylate. At each level, it's not a bad idea to do another very thorough search of everything that you're using. Perhaps, for example, you replaced a product in your house without rechecking the label, and now it has a forbidden ingredient added. If nothing bad turns up and your map hasn't changed, you may be inclined to raise your dosage.

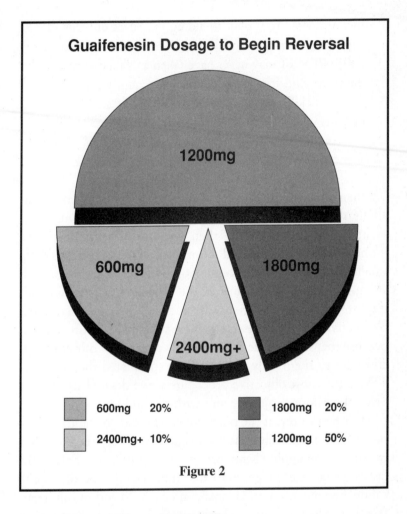

Guaifenesin Dosage to Begin Reversal

1200mg

600mg

1800mg

2400mg+

| | 600mg | 20% | | 1800mg | 20% |
| | 2400mg+ | 10% | | 1200mg | 50% |

Figure 2

Remapping While on Guaifenesin

Doctor L., I wanted to document my progress for you so you will have a reference point. You are the sort of open-minded physician who will be able to help many with this protocol. Your help in aiding me ferret out this illness has been invaluable. Had you not labeled it CFIDS/FMS I may never have taken a chance on trying the treatment. It is my hope that through my experience and your skill you will be able to help those among your patients who have suffered similarly.

—excerpt from a letter to her physician,
written by Gretchen P., South Carolina

We map our patients at every visit. Once we're more confident about their dosage, we can gradually stretch their appointments out—first to four, then six, and finally to twelve months. Their lumps and bumps should get progressively smaller, softer, or more mobile. Some of the larger ones, such as those at the hips or tops of the shoulders, will often split into smaller pieces. Patients have usually experienced some pain activity in the same areas where we palpate improvement, because that's where the action was. We put away our old maps and refer to them only after we have completed the new one. This is the most objective procedure we've devised to validate reversal without subjective and wishful thinking.

It is best to revisit the practitioner who did your initial mapping to keep the technique comparable. At every stage of your treatment, remapping is important, but especially once the early, fast-clearing areas are gone. At that time, changes become quite subtle, because fewer areas remain affected. To add to this, guaifenesin works much more slowly in certain types of tissues such as tendons and ligaments. These structures have low blood supplies, allowing only slower cleansing forces to penetrate.

You and your physician should agree on the frequency of mapping, choosing a schedule that's comfortable for both of

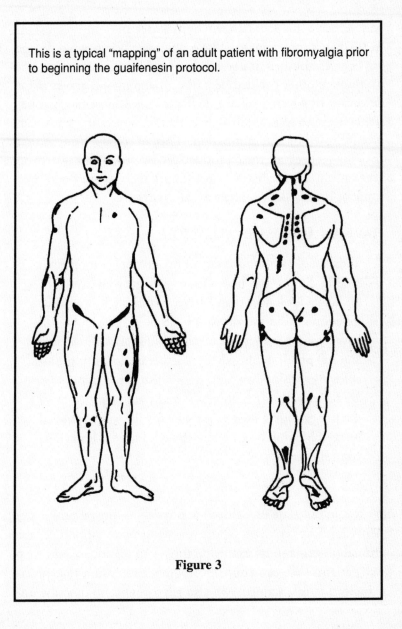

This is a typical "mapping" of an adult patient with fibromyalgia prior to beginning the guaifenesin protocol.

Figure 3

you. Once a map has shown initial clearing, any regression from that improvement will be obvious. When your dosage has been established, it doesn't change. Therefore, we must not overlook another decided benefit of mapping—it allows rapid detection of adverse salicylate effects. Since most blocked patients begin to feel rapidly worse, their deteriorating status can be confirmed by an examination. This, of course, requires that patients recheck all their products. We've used this system to great advantage for many years. That's the way we discovered some of the sneakier sources of salicylates.

HAVE AN ANNUAL EVALUATION

> Today marks my anniversary of my first full year on guaifenesin. I know you have a lot of patients who have been on guai a lot longer than I have, but to me it is a major milestone. I did not develop FMS overnight, and I still have a long way to go. Whenever I find myself in a cycle and full of self-doubts about whether or not your protocol works, I sit down and make a list of the things that are better with my health now, and I am surprised at all the things I list. I used to feel like my life was controlled by my FMS, but now I feel as though I have at least some control over it.
>
> —*Barbara C., Virginia*

By law, in our state of California, physicians must examine patients at least once a year before renewing a prescription. These annual or semiannual exams permit us to reevaluate and map our patients. We can confirm progress and ensure that previous clearing is sustained. We also get a chance to describe updated changes and warn of new products that might block previous gains. Thus, a checkup by your primary doctor provides important time for full evaluation of your general health.

Eventually almost all patients ask us how long they should continue taking guaifenesin after getting well. The answer to this question is simple. Guaifenesin only works when you're taking it. The treatment won't alter your genetic defect, which persists and, if unchecked, may cause your disease to resurface. It will not come back all at once, or even overnight, but it almost assuredly will return. Rather dependably, we found with our patients that the dose that caused their first reversal cycle is their dose for life if they choose to prevent rather than treat intermittently.

For some people, there's always a strong temptation to try lowering the dosage when they begin feeling better. If you increased your medication during the course of treatment just to speed up the reversal, lowering your intake to your original effective dosage may be advisable. But if you drop your dosage too low—to less than your therapeutic level—your fibromyalgia likely will come back. If you decide to try to lower the amount anyway, use a calendar and make notations about your various symptoms. If you see that you are losing ground and your symptoms are returning, resume your proper dosage and hold the line thereafter. After all, you're dealing with an unusually safe drug and can afford using a tiny amount more than absolutely necessary.

Did Something Else Sneak in When You Weren't Looking?

My most disturbing symptom was panic attacks. I would be overcome with a terrible feeling of impending doom. My hands would shake. I would be frantically afraid for no reason. Nothing I could think of would help. What finally helped was the hypoglycemic diet. Not once did I ever think that these attacks were from my blood sugar going wacky and that what I needed was to control my diet and thus control my blood sugar and thus ensure tranquility of mood.

—*F. W., Los Angeles, California*

When you have been officially diagnosed with fibromyalgia, you have another important item to discuss with your doctor. According to statistics tabulated from our practice of thousands, if you are a woman, there is approximately a 40 percent chance that you also have hypoglycemia, and an even greater chance of carbohydrate intolerance. It's imperative that you address this possibility before you finish your first consultation.

As we'll explain in detail in chapter 3, on hypoglycemia, there is no completely accurate blood test for this condition. The best way to decide whether or not you have this added burden is through incisive history questioning by your doctor. This can be a sticky issue. Many physicians aren't aware of the pitfalls in the standard five-hour glucose tolerance test used to diagnose hypoglycemia. Believe it or not, simple answers to a few astute questions are far more diagnostic. We'll develop this concept later.

You should be asked about two kinds of symptoms: the acute symptoms and the chronic ones hypoglycemia causes. Normally physicians begin questioning about the acute ones, because they're the easiest to identify. Acute symptoms generally occur within three or four hours after eating, and quite commonly during the night. They appear very suddenly and sometimes dramatically as horrifying panic attacks. Usually their onset is less startling and is accompanied by hunger, anxiety, hand tremors or inner shaking, sudden clammy sweating, and pounding or irregularities of heart rhythm (palpitations), often topped off with a pressurelike frontal headache. All of these may not occur at the same time in every hypoglycemic; they generally cluster in twenty- to thirty-minute episodes at specific intervals after eating too many carbohydrates.

The chronic symptoms are more generalized and do not provide such obvious diagnostic clues. They simply cruise somewhat steadily through your life no matter where your blood sugar stands. They don't totally derive from the drastic fall in sugar that produces the acute symptoms but arise from the systemwide, metabolic distress caused by repeated bouts of hypoglycemia.

Headaches are felt mainly in the front of the head as a dull pressure, especially when you've grabbed the wrong food or haven't eaten for a while. Fatigue, irritability, nervousness, flushing, impaired memory and concentration, tight muscles, and irritable bowel syndrome (abdominal pain, bloating, gas, and diarrhea) are among the most common of the chronic symptoms. If they appear when you're hungry and eating makes some of them go away, low blood sugar is the most likely culprit.

Even if you don't have *all* the symptoms we've listed, you may still be carbohydrate intolerant without full-blown hypoglycemia and would greatly improve on a restricted diet. This intolerance is best defined as having many of the chronic symptoms without the acute ones. Your doctor should review your diet and any relationship between what and when you eat, and your complaints. Clues arise from your food cravings, and from how you feel after consuming a large amount of carbohydrates.

If you're hypoglycemic or carbohydrate intolerant, you should begin our diet. This is the best diet we know of to control hypoglycemia. And it has been used successfully by many of our patients. Other low-carbohydrate diets are constructed primarily for weight loss or for increasing energy and are not designed specifically to control hypoglycemia or carbohydrate intolerance. Carefully read the pertinent hypoglycemia chapter in this book, and make a couple of copies of the diet. You may want one for your purse or wallet, and one for your refrigerator door. Before you eat anything, make sure it's listed on the diet. *You must follow the instructions strictly for two months before you begin to experiment with unlisted foods.*

If you intend to lose weight, you should talk to your doctor about following the strict diet outlined in chapter 5. Though it isn't better than the more liberal diet outlined in chapter 3 for controlling hypoglycemia, you can achieve two benefits at one time. When you've lost the weight you want, you're ready for weight maintenance. You may then add any of the foods from the liberal section.

If you're at a normal weight or underweight, the basic hypoglycemia diet (chapter 3) is a better choice for you. This less restricted format will help control your blood sugar so that you don't lose weight that will be hard to regain. Since carbohydrates are a culprit in weight gain, avoiding them too carefully will result in weight loss. It's important to eat enough of the listed vegetables, grains, fruits, and dairy products that you don't get too thin. Combining fats and carbohydrates usually prevents weight drop. Since you've heard repeatedly that it may be a good idea to avoid fats, this may be confusing in a book dedicated to improved health. We'll clarify the issue when we get to the discussions about cholesterol and blood fat levels.

If you're content with your weight and aren't carbohydrate intolerant, you still might feel considerably better by avoiding sugar and heavy starches. In our experience, because of their inherited energy blockade, fibromyalgics who do this often get a jump-start in energy for reasons we'll explain later on. You can try the diet for a month or two; if you've then noticed no benefit, discontinue it.

You'll have to carefully plan your menus at first. Shopping may be slow and a little laborious until you get the hang of the diet. You'll be delayed by reading listed contents, so allow extra time for scanning labels. We suggest carrying a magnifying glass in your purse with a copy of the diet. Pay special attention to the "Foods to Avoid Strictly" section when you're reviewing ingredients. It won't take very long before the process becomes second nature to you.

> At the end of the road you will find your life again. Is this not worth anything you have to endure? It is similar to the process of birth. At the end of the agony of labor you are gifted with a new life. The pain is forgotten in the joy. Press on, people. The reward is the most precious thing you can possess, your health. If you have your health you have everything you need. Nothing else compares as good health enables you to do whatever you desire in life.
> —*Kathleen Shuller, Panama City, Florida*

We're often asked by patients if they should start the diet before the guaifenesin, or vice versa. Our opinion is that it's best to start them both at the same time, marking a clear beginning to your new life. Guaifenesin's beneficial changes are slow compared to the dietary ones. Although the required change in metabolism may cause you to feel more tired and irritable for a few weeks, in about two months (assuming you haven't cheated) you will have accrued the benefits your new diet has to offer. For many, this is a substantial reduction in pain levels, and a corresponding surge in energy. It occurs at a crucial time, and encourages many a patient to continue on.

Chapter 1

Why We Focus on Energy and Where Did My Energy Go?

These are my symptoms in order of severity: extreme fatigue (sometimes I can hardly get out of bed). Sleeplessness and unrested sleep (no matter how much I need sleep—I sleep, wake up, sleep, wake up, et cetera all night). Feeling disconnected from my body, like I'm in a dream (this often scares me). Weak legs that feel heavy (it feels like I'm carrying something heavy in my hands and my legs are heavy). Neck, shoulder, and upper and lower back pain. Stiffness (mostly when I first wake up). Stinging, burning eyes. Pain around my eyes that feels like a sinus condition. Pain on top of my head. Forgetfulness. General achiness all over (I just feel like I'm sick). Tearfulness (because I feel so badly and I don't know what is wrong).

—*Marcia M. Los Angeles, California*

WHY FOCUS ON ENERGY?

If you have fibromyalgia, you know there's much more to it than just muscular pain. Most people with fibromyalgia agree:

"If it were only the pain, I could probably muck along some-how." It's the unrelenting adding and shifting of symptoms that eventually get you down. Headaches, brain fog, constipation suddenly yielding way to diarrhea, depression, backaches, anxiety, insomnia, apathy, or bladder pain—you never know what tomorrow will bring. And we're ignoring the oppressive fatigue. Oh yes, the overwhelming drop-dead fatigue that makes you feel like you've got to lie down when you're already lying down! Awful by itself, exhaustion on top of everything else that's wrong can make it impossible to cope with all of your other symptoms.

Most research and practicing physicians don't appreciate the extent of this total-body disaster unless they have fibro-myalgia themselves. When we speak to patient groups, we quickly get their attention by letting them know that we have it, too, and will never forget its punishing ways. What's it like? Fibromyalgia affects every cell in the body. Perhaps your doc-tor doesn't quite realize it, but you *know* it. All the time every minute of the day or night, something is wrong somewhere. Every fibromyalgic senses that his or her body just isn't right—sometimes each and every miserable part of it. Hair and nails don't grow without breaking, there's pain in strange places that can move around hourly, menstrual periods aren't regular or suddenly cause cramping, there's debilitating fatigue, devastat-ing headaches strike without warning, stamina is nil, sugar cravings are overpowering, and the resultant weight gain is de-pressing.

Physical complaints: debilitating *exhaustion*, severe *mus-cle pains* (especially shoulders, low back, neck, legs, arms), severe *joint pains* (shoulders, feet, hips, ankles, fingers), *headaches* (starting from the shoulders, up through the neck & around to front and sides of head), *sore throats, swollen glands* (neck, underarms, breasts), *nasal drip, water retention* (worse than usual), *clogged ears* (for several hours at a time), *worse allergies* than usual, *hypersensitivity* to bright lights and loud sounds, low-grade *fevers,* feeling *hot, flushing* red face, *insomnia:* 1. difficulty getting to & staying asleep 2. sleeping too long or too little 3. no matter how much sleep not rested, *mental disorientation* (difficulty concentrating and remembering), *agitation, irritability, depression, frequent tingling/numbness in extremities* (hands, feet, legs), *extreme discomfort* when lying or sitting in one position for long (*legs, arm pain*), *nausea, dizziness,* back-to-back *vaginal infections,* some *bladder infections, vaginal irritation and tears, pain with intercourse, weight gain* (approximately 15 pounds), *feeling hunger pains and ill* (after only a couple of hours of not eating), *mild gastro problems* (bloating gas, mild diarrhea, and occasionally constipation). Duration: 8/1999 to present. Became critical 4/2000.

—*actual patient intake form*

Most fibromyalgics have been conditioned to believe they're hypochondriacs and are perhaps stunned by the sheer volume of their own complaints. Then there's that certain look physicians sometimes give you during your symptom recital. Yet many fibromyalgic patients are among the most stalwart people we've met. For your vindication, published studies seem to bear this out. If you do a Medline search, you can read them for yourselves. Patients with chronic illnesses rate fibromyalgia more debilitating than rheumatoid arthritis. Many of our patients who have gone through cancer treatments say that, though they were challenged, frightened, and mentally and physically distraught, fibromyalgia, overall, is worse.

Fibromyalgics keep telling their doctors the same story. They don't have enough stamina to get through the day. That one deprivation is more frustrating than their pain. "No, Doctor, it's not mainly the pain that brings me in, though it would be nice if you could make it go away maybe just for an hour or two." They're usually too shy to add, "Please don't give me drugs that shove me deeper into my daily stupor. I'm really here because I'd like at least enough energy to start thinking clearly again."

Part of the problem is that all the parts of your body still work, but not at all well. You can walk, but not very far, and you certainly can't run. You think, but not very clearly. Obviously you remember your name, and what year it is, but your short-term memory can be very bad. You walk into a room and forget why you went in there. Maybe you can fall asleep, but then you wake up a lot and then lie there counting the hours as they tick by because you can't doze off. You may not be going bald visibly, but you're concerned by the poor quality of your hair and that it sometimes comes out by the handful. Your skin has patchy areas that have bumps or rashes of all descriptions. You get frustrated because you've always got a bunch of nagging complaints that don't *seem* connected. Oh, but they are! If you stop to think about it, what could the common denominator be for all these complaints? You should have no problem believing us when we say your body and its assorted parts just can't make enough energy.

Don't think in black and white. Certainly your body *can* make energy, but it is either *not doing it well* or doing it barely

enough to keep you alive. As a result, you have limited sta\
and feel older than your ninety-year-old antiquarian au.it.
Every cell in every system is functioning only marginally—just
hanging on. On the rare occasions when by sheer willpower
you force them into working full blast, you'll collapse and pay
for it for the next several days.

Since so many different tissues are affected, you find yourself vulnerable and susceptible to various pitfalls. Once fibromyalgia takes hold, people seem to suffer from more allergies
and catch infections as though bidding every bug welcome.
Heightened symptoms occur from odors, light, and sound, especially in women because their senses are already keener than
men's. Even minor things like colds seem to take forever to
heal. The reason is really quite simple: Recovering from such
things takes energy. When you're one of those fibromyalgic
people, where do you think you're going to get this? After all
these years, it's already perfectly clear to you that you can't
make enough energy. In the beginning, the body robs Peter to
pay Paul, but poor Peter is already in trouble, and beaten-
down Paul can't begin repaying the debt. There are simply too
many health problems all sucking on a very limited supply of
energy.

> People can't understand what having fibromyalgia feels
> like. . . . I finally came up with a combination of things
> anyone can understand. I tell them to imagine they have
> the flu and their belly is achy with gas and their head is
> pounding. Add to that they have not been able to sleep
> for a while and last night they didn't get any sleep at all
> so their mind is not working well. You also don't know
> when you're going to get any sleep. Now they have to

imagine that they were in a car accident and their whole body is stiff and sore. Next I tell them to imagine they have cinder blocks tied on their neck, waist, arms, and legs. Put all these things together at once and stay that way day and night for years. This is what fibromyalgia is. This is what I feel like all the time.

—*Shirley B., Louisiana*

In this chapter, we'll get into some details about the body's energy-production mechanisms. Most fibromyalgics have already heard a lot of technical jargon and too much mumbo-jumbo over the years. Every doctor seems to have a theory about what causes the illness, and you've heard of so many off-the-wall so-called cures. Your friends may beguile you with legends about a mountain-climbing former sicko who got well eating Brazilian jungle weeds. Your family cuts out articles from local papers and showers you with anecdotal tales they've heard from the cousin of a friend. You, too, have read and been told a lot of different things. What can you believe? Why us instead of them? Let's start at the beginning, then, and try to explain some basics to lead up to our solution for your problem. It seems logical that you should first understand what we think is assaulting your system before you accept our challenge to combat it.

I believe that I am functioning at about 50 percent of average capacity. I find holding down a part-time job extremely challenging. I am also having difficulty maintaining my weight and do not sleep well. I believe that the fatigue has become progressive. The pain has become

less acute but it has spread—that is, it is no longer local-
ized.

—*Sandra E., Los Angeles, California*

HOW DOES THE BODY MAKE ENERGY?

It's much easier to understand what's gone awry if you first
grasp how your body makes energy. The first thing that's
needed is fuel, and our cells grab up bloodborne molecules derived from what we eat in order to make it. Not all foods are
treated equally by the body, and their energy values are quite
different (we'll discuss this in more detail in chapter 3, on hypoglycemia). But basically, after digestion, breakdown products surge through the system. Cells take what they need and
direct this fuel to all kinds of hard-laboring enzymes. Various
internal compartments process each remnant into usable
snacks that are resurrected as energy. Huge amounts of high-
energy phosphates are also extracted and wedded to certain
proteins that should ideally empower anything your body
wants to do. All of this happens in thousandths of seconds,
staccatolike, until all required tasks are completed. When an
obstacle springs up anywhere along this series of biochemical
steps, however, you simply cannot produce the energy you
need.

We use 10 to 20 percent of our foodstuffs to create the
supportive structures of our tissues. These become the fabrics
that hold us together and contour our individually unique external appearance. Other frameworks shape the internal organs
that we can easily identify at a glance. The millions of cells
within those organs must have walls that allow them to lean on
their neighbors for maintaining their relative positions. Ever

smaller, often submicroscopic membranes define compartments housing the metabolic machinery inside those cells. There are even filamentlike highways where traffic moves along prescribed routes to deliver basic materials or finished products to and from those minuscule factories. All this fundamental construction work is needed to allow even the tiniest amount of movement. It also creates the dimensions enclosing billions of minuscule metabolic factories that seize the energy stored in the remaining 80 or 90 percent of our foods.

> To me pain is such a subjective experience that it's often difficult to know for sure whether I was feeling better or not. For a long time, observing the state of my kitchen was the method I used to tell how I was feeling. My kitchen had been in a constant state of turmoil (not to mention the rest of my house) for two years before I started the protocol. I was too tired to wash up after dinner, load and unload the dishwasher, et cetera. The sink and the counters were always cluttered with dirty dishes, and it seemed like the wastebasket was always full. Not a pretty picture. After a few months on guai I actually had the energy to take care of all those little tasks and clear my sink and counters. From then on, I used the state of my kitchen as a gauge—clean and tidy meant I was feeling pretty good . . . dirty and cluttered meant I was cycling hard. Now after three years, my whole house gets cleaned. . . .
>
> —*Nancy B., Cleveland, Ohio*

Like humans, all living things—plants and other animals—gobble up energy at a furious pace. Luckily for us and thanks to their chlorophyll content, plants can make their own energy directly from sunlight. They extract carbon dioxide floating in the atmosphere, much of which was exhaled by humans and the animals. Chemically trapping this simple gas, plants convert it into various carbohydrates. Thus, plants are the source of the sugars and starches that will, in turn, nourish the animals that consume them. It's a great relationship—at least for us at the top end of the food chain!

Humans generally don't eat only plants, though. We also eat other animals, a trait we share with them and with only a few carnivorous plants. Though it's a rather barbaric system, the benefits are positive for our survival, albeit one-sided. We're therefore blessed with two food sources, vegetable and animal. The latter provides most of our protein needs and the former, carbohydrates and fiber. Both are sources of fat. All our energy for motor activities, thinking, breathing, and healing comes from our successfully preying upon the other inhabitants sharing our planet. Let's look more closely at how our bodies convert these once living tissues into power.

Remnants of the three basic fuels—that is, fat, carbohydrate, and protein—are fated for destruction in energy-generating plants inside each cell, known as mitochondria. Every cell in the body has multiple generators and, depending on the tissue, may be quite densely populated with them. Here, wonderful concoctions are derived from the energy stores that nature instills into our foodstuffs. Gearlike enzymes working within the mitochondria process and restructure whatever is needed. Waste is produced but is expediently disposed of as two simple residues: water, and the gas carbon dioxide. From these magical activities, the currency of energy, adenosine triphosphate (ATP), is born.

The industrial prowess of a cell is second to nothing else we know, and it certainly meets strenuous demands. There is unrelenting wear and tear, much like what occurs with human-made machinery. As a result, a constant regeneration process goes on day and night. Essential chemicals must be imported for this reconstruction. Chromosomes use a lot of material while repeatedly dividing and creating new daughter cells. They must also direct all the cell's production lines. Eggs and sperms are generated and stuffed full of coded information in preparation for reproduction. All the while human arms and legs move, support, tug, or lift. Livers sort, store, or produce goods even while overseeing removal of toxins that periodically invade the system. Kidneys identify, purify, and purge the delivered by-products of metabolism, making instant determinations of what to save or excrete. Hair and nails grow, eyes blink, and hearts beat. Unlike the intestines, muscles, or bones, which are permitted intermittent, partial rest, the cells of the heart, brain, and blood are never awarded such luxury. Above all, the brain is continuously thinking and choreographing much of this biologic dance.

In every cell in our bodies, signals are coming in and out from every direction. These interconnections and functions are not luxuries. They are the very necessities for staying alive. This physiologic frenzy and perpetual activity requires energy. Most of the time cells rise to the challenge.

An Overview of Mitochondria, Your Biologic Power Stations (The Technical Stuff)

I have been hiding my chronic fatigue since I was seven. I was at that time diagnosed with "mono" and got better just as quickly and profoundly as I got sick, only to have it occur again and again until after the "mono" was long gone. My family quickly concluded that I was a malingerer that got sick when convenient to avoid family responsibilities. I quickly learned to tough it out and make hay while the sun shines because tomorrow I may need to spend the day in bed.

—*Roseanna, California*

Most structures inside cells were barely visible to early scientists, who only had primitive microscopes that provided very limited magnification. Additionally, the searching eyes peering down the tube had no idea what to expect. No precedent existed for something that had never before been seen. The barely distinguishable mitochondria appeared like a bunch of threads interlaced with granular bumps. Accordingly, the early microanatomists coined a new word using Greek derivations to describe these tiny bodies. *Mito* means "thread" and *chondro*, "granules" or "cartilage." The name stuck, but now we know it poorly describes the actual purpose and complex functions of these little organelles.

Mitochondrion is the singular form, which is rarely used. The reason for this is simply that there are so many in each cell. One muscle fiber may have anywhere from a few hundred to one thousand mitochondria. One unfertilized egg may contain up to five hundred thousand. That such numbers exist within single cells reveals their importance. Mitochondria are also widely varied: They come in different shapes and sizes and vary greatly from their cohorts. Some snuggle up close to different enclosures strewn about the cell, such as the nucleus and the endoplasmic reticulum where proteins are manufactured.

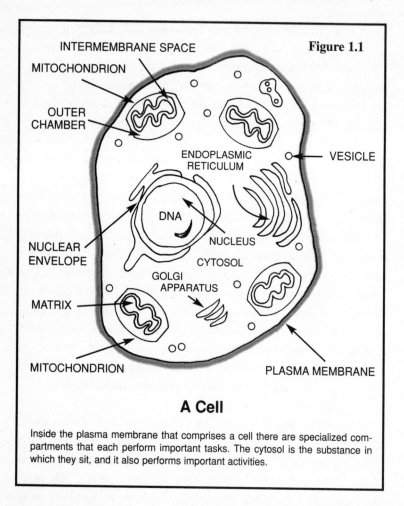

Figure 1.1

A Cell

Inside the plasma membrane that comprises a cell there are specialized compartments that each perform important tasks. The cytosol is the substance in which they sit, and it also performs important activities.

Others freely link up with fellow mitochondria and mutually digest information in some currently incomprehensible, biochemical language.

Today, scientists are finally able to peer into the depths of mitochondria. With new technology, they're no longer reduced to studying stained slides looking only at bits of totally dead and nonfunctional tissue. Researchers are no longer content with simply viewing structures and their anatomy. Newer techniques actually allow amplified spying into the chemical machinery while it's in action and very much alive. From these displays, even more startling findings keep emerging. We hope not to lose some of the marvelous intricacies by our simplifications, but at the same time we'll try to make a complexity more comprehensible.

> Fatigue was my middle name, and my friends after years of joking and ribbing me about falling asleep with twenty people in my living room and at every movie or theater event learned not to call me after 8:30 P.M. I have been on the protocol for about fifteen months and experience only intermittent fatigue. I still have a long way to go to get rid of the headaches, lower back pain, neck, shoulder pain, et cetera, but the progress is very freeing and gives me great hope for a completely normal life.
> —*M. Bailey, Fresno, California*

Mitochondria are really like franchised production kitchens that stir up the biologically tasteful, chemical soups necessary to meet all cellular nourishment needs. The broth originates with a roux of disintegrated food residues, mainly from carbohydrates and fats. These ingredients are further flavored with various minerals and spiced with the by-products of the chemical whirl itself. Enzymes heat and push the process to speed mixing and, in a few thousandths of a second, the concoction is ready. It is energy, and it's the same recipe imbibed throughout evolution by both plants and animals.

The whole process is carried out at electrifying speed. When there's a sudden need for action, invisible sparks actually fly rapidly around other cells. Try sprinting down the street and you'll sense the surge of energy you're expending. This spurt requires several physiologic procedures that must occur in an amazingly precise and prescribed order. Hundreds of chemical sequences are involved, each demanding cooperation from a matching enzyme. Awesome as it is to ponder this entire process, detailed chemical description is unnecessary in this text. For now, let's just look at the larger picture.

Mitochondria have two compartments, an inner and an outer chamber. Each has its own encircling membrane designed to keep out intruders. The outer wall interfaces with the rest of the cell and all its fluid contents. This membrane is relatively porous and lets in all kinds of compounds and chemical messages. Streams of various molecules and chemicals from all parts of the parent cell are allowed access. As you would guess, however, because of this lax security it's possible for undesirable and uninvited compounds to sneak in and snarl energy-generating mechanisms.

The inner wall is far more discriminating and protects the inner chamber, known as the matrix. This second room inside mitochondria is guarded by a formidable, electrified double wall that's similar to a security system, designed to protect the innermost chemical brain of the working cell. This core contains very delicate machinery that must be kept under constant surveillance and made safe from intrusive tampering.

Within the bastions of this inner chamber, several chemical steps are required to produce ATP, the currency of energy. If your body is functioning at a normal level, the powerful hy-

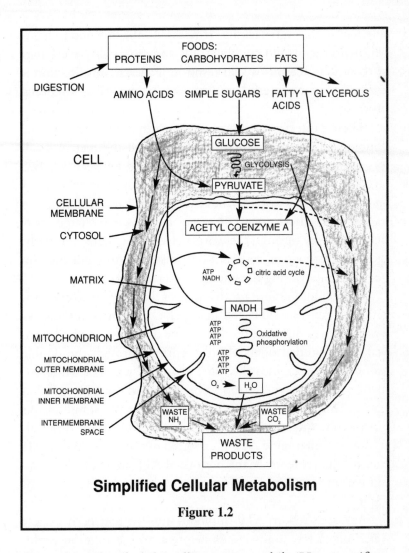

Simplified Cellular Metabolism

Figure 1.2

drogen ions that fuel the cells are very mobile. However, if excess cell baggage is present, energy formation ceases. A few paragraphs back, we mentioned that security in the little outside hall is glaringly lacking. If released into this outer chamber, hydrogen would readily escape and overacidify every part of the cell. Since this would result in its death, misdirection is prevented by a powerful security system comprised of special proteins.

These protectors promptly reattach hydrogen to the same double wall through which they just exited the matrix. Each ion sneaks back into the tiny space wedged between the two layers of the inner wall. In this space, the ion now encounters an entirely new set of enzymes that strip it naked—freeing up its one and only electron. Electrons are the same charged particles that flow through the world's electrical circuits. Similarly, they flow through all cells, not only disseminating information but also empowering the energy makers.

This combination of the proper ingredients comes together to generate ATP, and going clockwise or counterclockwise produces different results. In one direction, the hydrogen that was denuded of its electron sprints through the double wall directly back into the inner chamber, where it will eventually attract a new electron to become a whole hydrogen ion again. The energy of that same rotation gives simultaneous birth to one tiny morsel of ATP. Spin the rotor in the other direction and that same ATP is exported out to serve all the cell's energy requirements. Many pounds of ATP are made daily, because a huge amount of energy is needed everywhere, day or night.

As fast as reborn ATP implodes into the matrix, it usually waits only a few milliseconds before a reverse rotation explosively extrudes it right back out. It will be spent in widely distributed areas of the cell. Every function in the deepest recesses of your body depends on these exports. Nothing else can be used as a substitute.

Cashing in at the Energy Bank: ATP and ADP

> This year I was able to shop and prepare for Christmas all on my own. Last year I could barely drag myself through it and could not wait for my children to go back home. This year not only were my children here for nine days of celebration, but also our son brought home his new girlfriend for the whole time, too. We had a ball and I didn't miss a thing. I started a new job on January 4. Rolling out of bed and battling traffic was tough, but I love the work and the people exposure. It is not many hours a day, and I have to rest a day in between, but I am out and about and loving it.
>
> —*Gretchen P., South Carolina*

No single organ provides power to the entire human body. The beauty of decentralization is that every individual cell is involved in servicing its own requirements. This makes it impossible to shut down the body's entire energy supply at one time until death occurs. Even when many cells are damaged, remnant mitochondria within the injured system remain productive. They grind out extra ATP as best they can.

If only wounded, mitochondria will greatly slow their activity in order to survive. This reflects the body's prime directive: survival. Such slowing down allows the structure to remain viable, but leaves the body without surpluses. We've now arrived at the bottom line: *Chronic illness leaves the body with enough energy for basic functions only, with none to spare for the luxury of extra activities.*

If you've been patient enough to stick with us through this technical description, you probably have a better understanding of what causes fatigue. Biologic energy has a real chemical basis. It's not just some mysterious vapor that can't be measured. ATP energy is generated within actual factories in mitochondria. You may not have the same production capacity as some people. Believe it or not, there are probably some even less endowed than you. View this spread as a spectrum of possibilities. At one end are those energetic souls that need very little rest and bounce around everywhere doing more than ten others. There are also humans who barely hang on—appearing drugged, droopy-lidded, mustering every last ounce of energy just to sneeze. While we were not all equally gifted in the gene pool, whatever energy assets we once possessed can be recovered.

If you picked up this book and have read this far, you must suffer at least a modicum of energy deprivation. You're probably looking for an answer. Maybe you now understand more about why you're currently running on empty. If no one else has been able to help you, keep reading!

In this book, we'll explore some of the possibilities for your energy depletion. We can state right now that it certainly isn't due to lack of fuel. Fuel must be reaching the energy rotors of the mitochondria or you'd be dead. So we know that your fatigue is due to a shortage of ATP. If you don't have an acute or terminal illness, some chronic culprit is responsible for this theft. Fibromyalgia is one reason why you may be tired, but this disease also has many nasty collaborators.

We'll identify some of those common and major offenders in the ensuing chapters, and we'll tell you ways you can help to avoid them.

Chapter 2

Fibromyalgia *Means* Chronic Fatigue: Why This Disease Makes You So Darn Tired

The great thing about having fibromyalgia is that it explains everything wrong with me! Once I realized that, I was free from worrying about so many other maladies. My knees don't need to be replaced. I'll just wait two or three days and they'll be fine. I don't have carpal tunnel syndrome, it's just that I'm cycling in my sprained thumb. I don't have a slipped disc in my spine, it's just doing its fibro-thing. I've wondered if I've had rosacea, and all of the following cancers: bladder, colon, mouth, breast, and vaginal or bone. Amazingly, I do not have rheumatoid arthritis, lupus, Epstein Barr. I am not permanently insane, or prematurely senile. All of these maladies are *not mine,* and depending how strictly I followed my diet and took my guaifenesin I have perfect health. I just have to wait for it to transcend the latest iteration of its "cycle."

—*Claudia G., Eugene, Oregon*

Thirty-five million women, many men, as well as children of both sexes suffer with the serious energy warp that is fibromyalgia. Myriad others have been labeled with *chronic fatigue, candidiasis,* or other pseudonyms for what is the same debilitating condition.

If you're one of these sufferers, getting well probably seems beyond your grasp. Well, that's not necessarily so. Muster your strength and let's extend your reach. If you plan to repair your energy wheel, you can't very well ignore fibromyalgia. You'd certainly get something less than ideal results. In this and succeeding chapters, we're going to show you how to achieve a well-balanced wheel from the raw material your genes have provided you. It's all about integrated function.

With some illnesses, significant improvement can be achieved through a single medication or treatment despite only token patient cooperation. Unfortunately, fibromyalgia and most of its related disorders are not among these. To regain a healthy version of yourself, some demands will be made of you; you can't just sit there passively. You'll have to acquire some knowledge and expertise about your current condition. Armed with new resources, you will find it possible to stimulate a far more energetic you. Even then, however, you'll have to remain dedicated and remain alert to avoid future damage to your repairs.

WHY DO WE THINK THE PROBLEM IS ENERGY?

I went to go see a diagnostic specialist about a three-hour drive from my home. I wanted to go see him because of the twenty-eight doctors I had already seen who told me: "Good news!" (Really?) "You're fine." (That's not good news!) "There's nothing wrong with you." (Oh, no! You're stupid too!) "If there was something wrong with you it would be in your head." (You've got to be kidding me. I think you're the crazy one.) "So get some counseling." (More? Again?) "Get off your butt." (Trust me, I would love to.) "Avoid stress." (I wish.) "Drink lots of fluids." (I spend more on water than I do on food.) "And get some rest." (I sleep twenty hours a day, isn't that enough?)

—*Chandra S., Marina, California*

The wide range of organs and tissues affected by fibromyalgia should alert you to ask, "What kind of illness could affect so many systems of the body? Why can't we find any abnormality on diagnostic tests? Why doesn't it go away with medications or exercise? Why don't dietary changes help?" These are some of the issues that physicians and patients alike address and ponder. Even those of us who have studied fibromyalgia for years don't agree on the answers. Luckily, we do agree at least on the questions.

As we've mentioned in many previous writings, there are so many varying theories on what fibromyalgia is that it makes it very difficult to get a diagnosis—much less suitable treatment. Lacking uniformity within the medical community on the nature of fibromyalgia, let's offer our own theories. We offer no apology for a lifetime of observations on this disease. We present firsthand evidence gathered from several thousand fibromyalgia patients. It also includes facts gleaned from our own battles with fibromyalgia; yes, from both authors and our families. We're certainly on a mission and plan to share our knowledge with you. Perhaps you'll agree that what we have to say does make sense from a physiologic and biochemical perspective. There are still some physicians and patients who don't believe we're right in bunching chronic fatigue, chronic candidiasis, vulvar pain, and myofascial pain into a single disease, yet you'll see the similarities between fibromyalgia as we describe it and these other so-called syndromes. At one time, it certainly was accepted as gospel that chronic fatigue and fibromyalgia were two different entities. These days, however, it's a generally accepted concept that they're just different presentations of the same disease.

If we could rename this larger disorder, ill designated as fibromyalgia, we would choose the term *dysenergism syndrome* (faulty energy). It's no secret that a name that means only "pain in the muscles and fibers" describes only the tip of the iceberg. We really do need a name to better reflect both patient fatigue and cellular failure as reflections of the same basic metabolic problem. Our patients comment that they can't summon enough energy to go through the basic routine of daily chores. *Anergism* (absence of energy) would effectively describe this lack of vigor in both the struggling patient and the weakened cells. For the purposes of this book, however, we'll stick with the name *fibromyalgia* because it's the commonly accepted term for this disorder. We'll use it to refer to all of the various syndromes, symptoms, and orphan syndromes named above.

Our treatment is designed to restore energy production by releasing the body from a biochemical blockade. When this is accomplished, the symptoms of the illness will gradually reverse and finally disappear. Patients who've felt themselves aging too rapidly should revel in the joy of rejuvenation.

The Symptoms of Fibromyalgia

By and large, fibromyalgia symptoms may be grouped into the following categories: cerebral, musculoskeletal, gastrointestinal, dermal, genitourinary, and eye-ear-nose-and-throat. There are also a few other isolated problems that don't fit easily into any classification. If we look at the range of symptoms that fibromyalgics experience, then it is little wonder their bodies are so exhausted. In our first book, we gave each of these groups its own, individual chapter. You may wish to refer to it if you want more detailed information.

Cerebral: Fatigue, irritability, nervousness, depression, impaired memory and concentration (popularly known as "fibrofog"), apathy, frequent awakening during the night, nonrestorative sleep, blurred vision, dizziness, and headaches (often labeled migraines because of their intensity).

Musculoskeletal: Widespread, aching pain and stiffness in muscles, tendons, and ligaments, which is often worse upon awakening. Pain intensity varies and presents in many forms such as throbbing, burning, stabbing, stinging, grabbing, or combinations of these. Numbness of the extremities or face and tingling almost anywhere arise from spastic structures pressing on nearby nerves. Temporomandibular joint involvement causes difficulty in chewing or sometimes excruciating facial and head pain. Neck lesions produce the most complaints, including headaches. Muscles often display repeated little twitches. The restless leg syndrome makes it impossible to find a comfortable spot for rest. Patients also complain of feelings like electrical impulses shooting through their muscles, and of an exhaustive general weakness.

Dermal: Crawling sensations, itching, acne, dry skin, rashes (many varieties), burning, and sometimes swollen and hot-itching palms and soles of the feet. Patients often have brittle nails, poor hair quality, as well as a slightly pungent and irritating perspiration.

Gastrointestinal ("fibrogut"): Irritable bowel syndrome that includes gas, pain, bloating, constipation alternating with diarrhea, and sometimes nausea or hyperacidity with acid reflux.

Genitourinary: Vulvodynia, which includes vulvitis and vestibulitis (raw, irritated, burning vaginal lips or deeper areas), vaginal spasms, burning discharge, increased menstrual and uterine cramps, painful intercourse (dyspareunia), repeated bladder infections, pungent, concentrated urine, and chronic interstitial cystitis.

Eye-Ear-Nose-Throat: Eye irritation or dryness and burning tears, blurred vision, excessive or sticky discharge with morning "sand," sudden imbalance or dizziness, vertigo (spinning due to middle ear involvement), strange sounds (particularly ringing, or tinnitus), postnasal drip, chronic nasal congestion, foul or scalded (sometimes transient) metallic tastes, painful or cut tongue, persistent sore throats without infection.

Miscellaneous: Buckling knees when walking, low-grade fevers, Raynaud's phenomenon (blanching of fingers exposed to cold), increased allergies, and sensitivity to light, sounds, and odors.

Much has been discussed and written about fibromyalgia. Despite this, it too often goes unrecognized. Some physicians still deny its existence. Books are rapidly accumulating on the subject, and though most define the illness rather well, rare are those that offer anything beyond coping. Our own two, *What Your Doctor May* Not *Tell You About Fibromyalgia* and *What Your Doctor May* Not *Tell You About Pediatric Fibromyalgia,* are already part of the fibromyalgia library. They go into sufficient detail that we can more quickly review the disease in this book. We'll outline our clinical experience and hopefully anticipate questions you might have.

So what is fibromyalgia? If we break the name down, you'll quickly understand how little of the illness the word describes. *Fibro* refers to the fibers located in the various connective tissues and *myo,* to muscles. The suffix *algia* denotes pain. Recombining the syllables suggests an entity that is manifested by pain in fibers and muscles. *Fibromyalgia* is thus a misnomer— a fact that was likely understood by those who named it about twenty years ago. This term better reflected some glaring aspects of the disease than did the previous designation, *fibrositis,* which implied nonexistent inflammation. Neither is really better than the older name, *rheumatism*—except that, perhaps, rheumatism is what you expect your grandmother to have. Yet all are somewhat apt since they at least suggest musculoskeletal aching and stiffness. Each term almost totally misses the hallmark of this disease, which is why we offer our replacement, *dysenergism,* introduced above. Energy deprivation is almost universal among patients as a common denominator of what is technically known as the fibromyalgia syndrome.

If you grew up in the Sahara Desert, you might be tempted to believe that the whole world is covered with sand. That is somewhat like our perception of normal body function. If you've suffered the symptoms of fibromyalgia, you might actually assume your fatigue is the price paid for simply existing. You will probably think everybody feels that way. It may take you some time to realize what normal is, and how many of your complaints are linked to this one illness. Let's take a moment to review how they group into the common syndromes partially accepted by the medical profession.

Central Nervous System: This is like a real brain sprain. Most common are: fatigue, irritability, nervousness, depression, apathy, listlessness, impaired memory and concentration, anxieties, and suicidal thoughts. Insomnia is sometimes the inability to get to sleep but more often it is repeated and prolonged awakenings during the night. Frequent rousing is usually secondary to the rapidly cumulative discomfort of lying even for a few minutes in any one position. This evokes a nonrestorative rest profoundly reflected by daytime somnolence. Fears of premature Alzheimer's disease are fostered and nurtured by repeated cognitive impairment. They're certainly augmented by a frequent loss of awareness such as driving directly past familiar destinations and ending up in remote surroundings.

Musculoskeletal System: Aches, pains, and generalized morning stiffness spring from multiple affected muscles, tendons, ligaments, and joints. More common locations are in the shoulders, neck, hips, knees, inner and outer elbows, wrists, chest, and segments of or the entire back. Previous operative or injured sites are often preferentially affected. Less appreciated is the discomfort from spasms involving similar but deeper tissues within the chest, abdomen, or pelvis. Calf or foot cramps seem more common during the night. Erratic numbness or tingling often strikes fingers, toes, face, or any part of the body.

Irritable Bowel Syndrome: Among its synonyms are leaky gut, spastic colon, and mucous colitis. Also experienced are nausea, often in brief but repetitive waves, indigestion and acid reflux, deep aching or hard pain, gas, bloating, cramps, and constipation alternating with diarrhea that is sometimes accompanied by mucus in the stools.

Genitourinary Syndrome: Pungent urine, frequent urination, bladder spasms, burning on urination (dysuria), repeated infections (cystitis), or interstitial cystitis occur. The term *vulvodynia* (vulvar pain syndrome) includes deep vaginal contractions, labial itching, and irritation of the inner vaginal lips (vulvitis) or tissues surrounding the opening (vestibulitis). All are accompanied by painful intercourse (dyspareunia). These symptoms so closely mimic yeast infections that they're frequently diagnosed incorrectly. The distinguishing clue is the absence of the typical cottage cheese discharge. Menstrual uterine cramping often occurs even after bearing children. Deep muscular spasms may cause diffuse pelvic pain and are readily felt on pelvic examination. Most symptoms of fibromyalgia are worse during the premenstrual week.

Dermatologic Syndrome: Itching is common with or without the various rashes: scaly skin, hives, isolated red blotches, tiny pebbly bumps (red or clear), blisters, eczema, seborrheic or neurodermatitis, acne, and rosacea. Nails are brittle and often chip or peel steadily or sporadically. Hair has broken ends, is of poor quality, and falls out prematurely, often combing out in bunches. There may be intense burning or coldness of the skin, a supersensitivity to touch, crawling, prickling, or vibratory sensations, and often flushing with or without sweating. Red, burning, or itchy palms and soles are difficult to relieve. Some patients suffer dermal hyperreactivity by displaying linear welts that reproduce any figures inscribed on their skin using a fingernail or blunt object (dermatographia). Quite common and familiar, Raynaud's phenomenon evokes the sudden appearance of dead white fingers upon exposure to cold. Easy bruising is present in the vast majority of women, often appearing without apparent trauma.

Eye-Ear-Nose-Throat: Dry eyes occur, or the reverse, excessive watering with sticky tears that may evaporate during the night, leaving "sand" in the corners of the eyes. Intermittent visual blurring is frequent, as are burning, red, or itching eyes and eyelids. The lids may abruptly start fluttering due to repetitive contractions (blepharospasm).

The ears join in with brief hums, fluttering, or swishing sounds, but more often there's only a transient, high-pitched ringing. When such sounds are coupled with dizziness, Ménière's syndrome is often diagnosed. Dizziness or simply an awkward imbalance permits stumbling into furniture or doorjambs. Vertigo usually occurs when suddenly turning the head, especially when lying down. It is an alarming spin that forces grabbing on to the bed or any nearby, stable object.

Nasal congestion and postnasal drip together help create bad taste and breath. Reflective of excessive mineral content in salivary discharges, sudden metallic surges are tasted. The entire mouth may feel scalded and help create the offensive tastes. The tongue may hurt as though paper-cut, and its edges feel burned or sandpapered. Repeated open sores may also develop, suggesting herpes but on the wrong surfaces.

Miscellaneous Symptoms: Several symptoms do not easily fit into any of the above syndromes. Headaches may be accompanied by visual aberrations as well as nausea and vomiting; if severe enough, they're invariably diagnosed as migraines. Buckling knees even without pain may provoke instability or actually induce falling. There may be significant weight gain, low-grade fever, and heightened susceptibility to infection. The majority of our female and some of our male patients suffer an increased sensitivity to light, sounds, chemicals, or odors. Such challenges sometimes do more than simply irritate by inducing headaches, nausea, or severe nasal congestion.

Allergic reactions are often facilitated and manifested by hay fever or asthma. Palpitations are experienced as a rapid or forceful heartbeat and flip-flop sensations. Sudden water accumulation, especially during attacks, may range from two to four pounds. Its sequel is morning eyelid and hand puffiness that yields to progressive gravitational edema (swelling) of the lower legs toward day's end. The skin is uncomfortably stretched from within, resulting in the annoying restless leg syndrome.

AN OVERVIEW OF WHAT'S GOING AWRY WITH YOUR ENERGY

> Today I scrubbed a floor, prepared the house for the carpet cleaners, and took a brisk walk. Thank you.
> —*Dorothy M., Tempe, Arizona*

It is almost universally true that fibromyalgics suffer a marked loss of their former energy reserves. Patients are not restored by the pseudo-sleep they get each night. They remain tired despite frequent resting and are exhausted by even the simplest daytime activities. Fairly long respites usually appear in the early stages. Cyclic deterioration is likely, however, and eventually only bad days remain, interspersed with even worse days. Energy fades and can be fleetingly retrieved only by heroic efforts. Empowering even a minuscule task requires a gargantuan appeal to willpower.

When we began working on this book, one thing surprised even the two of us who work with fibromyalgia patients all day. Of course we knew from experience that fibromyalgics complain about being tired. We've tabulated our own statistics for about five years now, and they show that 99 percent of the patients who come into our office complain of deadening fatigue, as well as pain. What was surprising when we started to review our patients' charts, reading the medical history forms they'd filled out prior to their first appointment, was that, contrary to the impression you get from published articles, more patients complained about fatigue than pain. In other words, when asked about symptoms, patients will of course respond yes to the question about pain, and yes to the question about fatigue. But when asked to list their complaints, more often than not the first answer was "exhaustion."

There is abundant scientific evidence concerning the lack of energy in fibromyalgia. We made reference to some of these published studies in our previous books. These technical papers are often difficult to grasp even by people versed in medical sciences. We're avoiding the temptation to interpret these or newer data in a book primarily aimed at nonprofessionals.

The ensuing paragraphs are intended to satisfy your curiosity concerning how we evolved our treatment protocol. The theory that follows is based upon our experience and a synthesis of data gleaned from various biochemical research. Please remember that theories are only educated suppositions. What really counts is that we have an effective treatment for this illness and have successfully treated thousands of patients.

The body draws its energy from the mitochondria in each of its tiny cells. They are wondrous factories that cater to the needs of all living organisms. Regardless of their specialty, they have the ability to create thousands of enzymes, hormones, chemicals, structures, or genes. No exceptions are the nerve cells and connecting filaments that, like our home wiring, electrify the entire system. Hormonal surges are evoked from endocrine glands in response to their own particular set of stimulators and join the nerve endings in their cell-goading action. Most tissues need this bipartisan leadership to fulfill designated functions. Cells stop or start upon command and respectfully fill orders for their metabolic products. In further compliance, they ultimately export their wares for local or systemic distribution and consumption.

There's really an astounding amount of work to be done. Muscles are made up of cells that must labor heavily with every movement we make. The brain never quite totally rests. Its cells cannot just sit back totally dormant; they must perform too many routine functions simply to remain viable. There's a constant flow of incoming information that must be processed at all times. Day and night it thinks, dreams, and continues to keep in touch with the rest of the body. The skin, nails, and hair grow, and must at times be shed. This is an ongoing process even while digestive juices and enzymes are formed, packaged, and shipped to an encounter site with incoming fuel, the foods we eat. There is ample employment for every bodily system even when we're seemingly resting and doing nothing. On top of all of this, there is a fundamental rent that must be paid just for being alive. This sum is extracted from us second by second even during our sleeping or most sedentary moments. Altogether, they comprise our basic energy budget, the amount of energy we must spend just to stand still, cough, or perform any activity.

There is also much wear and tear in everyday living. With so much hard work to do meeting external demands, cells are always in need of repair. Their structures and assembly lines must be very well maintained. As we have seen, within each cell are a series of little power stations designed to provide the refined fuel we need to meet every contingency. They are the mitochondria we discussed in chapter 1, and they are chemically and electrically oriented to burn food residues through a set of chemical reactions called oxidation. Thus is born ATP, the currency of energy, which must be harnessed for almost any basic cell function.

There are various limitations placed upon how much energy we can maximally produce; some are, for example, genetic. We all have inherited different capacities, but the process of making energy is the same in all of us. To add to that, our cells also have storage systems where they hold reserves, and the raw material needed to produce more energy at the ready.

Now think back to the formidable list of symptoms of fibromyalgia we outlined above. Begin with the brain and the nervous system. Compile in your mind the gross energy expenditures required just to experience fatigue, stress, and pain. Remember the fact that the chemical signals allowing your brain to know there's an aching or throbbing pain somewhere must be manufactured. It takes a lot of energy to make these traveling messengers. Add this to the cost of nerve impulses that are generated for both external and internal communications. All these requests must be converted into electric currents the brain can interpret. It even takes energy to suffer emotionally.

If you're a sufferer of the disease, fibromyalgia is just exactly as you've described to your doctors. You experience overwhelming fatigue and there seems no ample reason for it. Not only do you feel tired, but your most severely affected cells are equally exhausted. Their inherent expenditures are the fundamental reason why you have no energy. They're constantly warning you, even screaming that you must stop, sit, and rest because "we, the cells just can't go any farther." It's the unrelenting energy deprivation that drives so many systems to fail. One section or another may occasionally rise to meet the metabolic challenge, but it soon recoils from duty when its own energy supply nears depletion. Another adjacent group of cells may step in to take up the slack, but they, too, will quickly falter for the same reason. There is never zero energy—that would result in death. Cells have a strong survival instinct, and when threatened with severe shortages enter a semihibernation mode using just enough energy to stay alive. They, and you, then have no energy left for other tasks that are deemed less important than survival.

Throughout every moment of your life, every part of your body works at all times to some degree. As we've stated above, this is true even when your body is at rest. Even in hibernation, cells cannot suspend all activity; each must maintain a small level of metabolism just to assure its survival. Since each system must provide for higher stress demands at different times, energy is quite variably expended. It all depends upon what challenge your body is dealing with at any given moment. We're trying to make it obvious to you that fibromyalgia has to be the result of a bodywide power depletion. Only one structure could let you down so drastically, and it has to be at the most fundamental, intracellular level. We point directly at mitochondria that, if not the prime culprits, at least seriously aid the failure. After all, they're the only structures that can create energy.

We were not born with the symptoms of fibromyalgia. Even though some patients tell us that they were born tired, in reality it takes time to develop the syndrome's hallmarks, and they occur at different ages in different people. We've seen three sets of identical twins who all developed fibromyalgia, though not quite at the same time. Each one presented with slightly different complaints and physical findings. From these facts, we can extrapolate the likelihood that patients are not born with any particular structural defect. Otherwise, identical twins would have identical aberrations.

We promised not to belabor incomprehensible technical data, so we won't. Let's simply state that we believe fibromyalgia to be an inherited illness, for several reasons. The foremost evidence is something we've seen with our own eyes: thousands of patients we've treated who had history of fibromyalgia in their family trees. We believe the genetic aberration is a defect in a kidney protein, probably an enzyme, which permits a minuscule but inexorable and daily retention of phosphate. Initially, the bones are very adept at tucking away such accumulations. When that capacity is overrun, as it eventually is, other structures must take up the excess. Ultimately, the accumulation is reflected in most cells, but particularly in the most active ones—the brain and the muscles.

Excess phosphate cannot enter cells arbitrarily. The body's goal is always balance, and each phosphate carries two negative charges. Since phosphate entering the cell would adversely tilt the electrical balance, it must be buffered. In steps calcium, with two positive charges—a perfect sort of molecular soul mate. Overabundant phosphate inside the cell blocks energy formation but doesn't cause the contraction of muscles, tendons, and ligaments that we invariably find when examining patients with fibromyalgia; calcium is the culprit responsible for this. It has prominent functions within all cellular units. It isn't bashful; it intrudes into almost all the body's nooks and crannies, dictating the duration and extent of the workload. When calcium lingers too long or refuses to leave, overtime labor is exacted. Calcium demands unrelenting work and eventually drives the affected cells to exhaustion. Excess phosphate in mitochondria slows the formation of ATP, which provides energy. This is all well-known biochemistry. It's this combination that makes fibromyalgia low energy, all work, no play, and no rest! Excess calcium drives the cell into continuous action, and excess phosphate makes the formation of energy needed for that action nearly impossible.

No other explanation fits the complete exhaustion of fibromyalgia. No other theory even begins to explain the connections among so many symptoms. There's considerable supportive research validating our stance. Energy deprivation due to faulty production and overutilization explains the entire illness. It's true that memory impairment is connected to chipping fingernails, rashes, bladder problems, and an irritable bowel. Stiffness, aches, and pains are likewise interrelated due to muscles, tendons, and ligaments that keep working day and night. Unfortunately, many clinicians are ignoring the neatly packaged evidence so astutely presented by their patients.

The symptoms and findings of fibromyalgia are caused by a lack of ATP. Luckily, a rationing system is instituted, conserving energy for the most vital organs so that no damage is sustained even though you are miserably ill. Obviously, the aim of treatment should be to restore energy to all affected cells. We must relieve the phosphate blockade and allow mitochondria to produce energy unimpeded. The ATP produced will first provide energy to the healthier cells, allowing them to purge themselves of accumulated debris. They in turn will help restore function and lend a hand to the remaining sick ones. When each system gets back on-line, the disease miraculously disappears.

HYPOGLYCEMIA, FIBROMYALGIA'S KNOCKOUT PUNCH

> That day I ran around making phone calls and announcing the good news to everyone. I was sick! I had something! A real disease with a real name and actual medical journal articles written about it! Some people probably thought I was crazy to be happy about such a diagnosis but they didn't know the hell I had been through. The persistent pain. The fatigue. The frustration of dealing with unknowing doctors.
>
> —*Michelle F., Palos Verdes, California*

We earlier warned that a large number of fibromyalgics suffer from hypoglycemia (low blood sugar) and carbohydrate intolerance for some very sound metabolic reasons. Insulin, as we'll discuss more fully in chapter 3, is released every time we eat carbohydrates. Some people produce too much of it. One of the prime functions of insulin in the body is to drive glucose into cells—but glucose doesn't enter alone. It drags phosphates with it. And as we've seen, excess phosphates in the cells of fibromyalgics is already the problem! Among the tissues most responsive to insulin are muscle cells, and they can be forced to accept inordinate amounts of phosphate. Insulin also signals certain kidney cells to reabsorb some phosphate that was scheduled for elimination in the urine. It stands to reason, then, that those with carbohydrate cravings or hypoglycemia will feel better if they follow the dietary restrictions we'll examine just ahead. Though no specific diet is needed for fibromyalgia, getting rid of the wide fluctuations of blood sugar will allow a surge of energy, and a lessening of both pain and the clouded mind we recognize as fibrofog. Irritable bowel is another symptom cluster that responds at least partially to the hypoglycemic diet.

If you're not sure where you stand regarding the blood sugar issue, be sure to read the next chapter carefully. If you're a fibromyalgic with hypoglycemia or strong carbohydrate cravings, be careful. Although fibromyalgia will yield to guaifenesin, dietary factors may be critical to whether you feel much better, despite the improvement on your body maps.

THERE IS HOPE

But I do remember the love and support from my family and friends, my boss and coworkers, my wonderful fiancé who would not let me give in to fibromyalgia. I remem-

ber how scared I was when I tried the guaifenesin protocol because I was afraid to get worse before I got better.
But I will never forget the first day I woke up and had *no*
pain and *no* fatigue. It was a joyous day . . . I knew I was
going back to work, I knew I was going to be able to do
all those things that so many people take for granted like
going grocery shopping or walking the dog.

—*Rachel*

As we've stated previously, our theories evolved only after realizing we had an effective treatment for fibromyalgia. What you
really care about is how to get rid of the disease. The preceding discussion of symptoms and energy formation was mainly
a preparation for what you'll read—and deal with—ahead.
Even this sketchy familiarity should help you grasp the logic of
our protocol. Now let's turn to how to make you feel better by
allowing your body to make the energy it needs.

Previously, we had some success treating fibromyalgia with
four older medications. All had been amply researched, and
their chemical impact well recognized. Two of them are still
available and remain effective for treating fibromyalgia. We
abandoned them not because of their failings, but for their potential side effects. Our previous knowledge made it easier for
us to appreciate the greater efficacy of our fifth drug. It's also a
very old medication with an unbelievable safety record. We
now use it almost exclusively with our patients: guaifenesin.

Guaifenesin seems ridiculous to some practitioners because it's marketed as a mucus-clearing agent. Mucus is certainly not an obvious component of fibromyalgia. We're quick
to agree, and it's true that we are promoting a new indication
for its use. Based on our experience, we endorse it as the most

powerful and safest medication we've found to date for reversing fibromyalgia. And the benefit of using a drug that's been on the market for so many years is that we know it's safe for long-term use, and we know that despite many years of use, no serious side effects have been reported.

It's true that guaifenesin is classified as an expectorant, one of a few compounds that stimulate mucus-producing cells. This is why it is compounded into many brands of cough medicines. For more than twenty years, it's been manufactured as a long-acting, 600 mg. tablet more easily handled than liquid preparations. In July 2002, because of the drug's safety record, the FDA granted one manufacturer a patent to produce guaifenesin over the counter in both 600 mg. and 1200 mg. strengths. The brand name for this new product is Mucinex. It is generally used by patients with chronic sinusitis, bronchitis, asthma, and lung diseases. Twenty-four hundred milligrams per day is standard dosing for such respiratory problems. Since it's designed for sustained action, two tablets are taken in the morning and two more twelve hours later. The majority of fibromyalgia patients need only about half that amount.

To give you an idea of the safety enjoyed by the drug, let's review the toxicity studies done in animals. No significant side effects were reported at 5,000 mg. per kilo in rats. That is equivalent to a 130-pound woman ingesting almost five hundred tablets all at one time. The parent bark extract of guaifenesin, guaiacum, was in use more than four hundred years ago and, as a great surprise to us, mainly for "rheumatism." No significant side effects were reported, and it's actually still being manufactured in that form.

Guaifenesin works by helping the kidneys increase their

excretion of various compounds. Because phosphate excesses fit the bill as the primary cause of fibromyalgia, we'll focus on that substance—for now. Please keep in mind that phosphate is only the theoretical culprit. We've measured a surge in urinary phosphate excretion before and after in a study using the older drug probenecid, and have repeated that experiment with guaifenesin. Kidneys have special sites, in the tubules, dedicated to the maintenance of phosphate balance. They accomplish this by either retaining or excreting phosphate according to signals they interpret. Guaifenesin almost certainly enters the scene at this special location.

Increasing urinary excretion of anything will usually decrease blood levels of that substance. It is our premise that the augmented phosphate excretion induced by guaifenesin removes the excess from the bloodstream. That, in turn, creates a siphoning effect on the accumulations hidden in various body fluids and affected tissues. Where renal retention once forced a backwash that ultimately resulted in cellular excesses, creating an opposite "imbalance" totally reverses the direction of the illness. Tissues can't chemically tolerate having an imbalance with the surrounding fluids, including blood, because it's physiologically unsound. Guaifenesin, like our four previous medications, simply creates a new equilibrium; an unbalanced equation is normalized. Simply stated, an outflow of phosphate replaces the previous inflow from retention. Once adversely impacted kidney enzymes are restored, full body function can be restored.

Many people ask why biopsies of fibromyalgic muscle tissues show no microscopic abnormalities. They surmise that excess calcium and phosphate should leave a visual trace. Yet this isn't so. When salt crystals are dropped into a glass of warm water, they can no longer be seen. Sodium and chloride are still present, but in an altered state. We say the salt is dissolved. Their individual electrified particles, or ions, are invisible. It is the same for the ions of calcium and phosphate. However, if we simply keep adding more table salt or calcium phosphate, we'll eventually have to add more water to keep the crystals in solution. The excess phosphates retained by fibromyalgic kidneys force retention of their traveling companion, calcium. In turn, they express their thirst by dragging water into cells, keeping the ions from crystallizing. Neither free ions nor water is seen under a microscope. Nevertheless, excess tissue water bloats and raises intracellular pressure. Swelling impacts nerve endings and creates pain. We can point out the effects as the lumps and bumps of fibromyalgia.

As we've seen, the reversal process begins when the accumulations are pulled out of affected cells. Water plays a very big, if underappreciated, role in this process. It's the moving force that helps eliminate excess phosphate and calcium. Guaifenesin simply prompts a reversal tide for unwanted phosphate that poses no threat to essential cellular function. During treatment, urine output fluctuates depending upon the need to hold water for dilution or expel it for excretion.

Illnesses generate complaints because they cause malfunction. Symptoms are the body's screams that something is wrong. Unfortunately, there are no treatment shortcuts. During reversal, recent symptoms are revisited, as eventually are older ones. The cleansing process is greatly accelerated, though—up to six times faster than it took to accumulate the deposits. Just as the illness developed in cycles during depositing phases, purging replicates aches and pains during extrac-

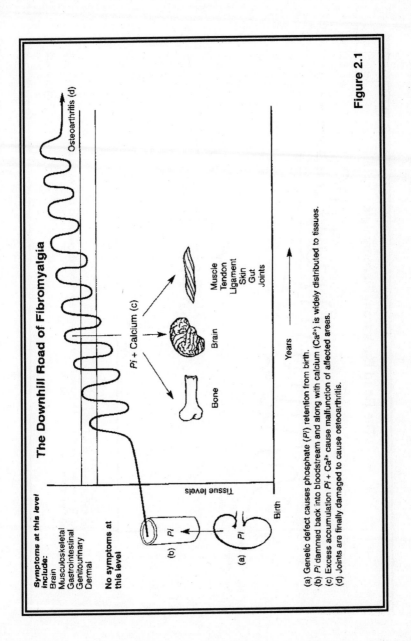

The Downhill Road of Fibromyalgia

Osteoarthritis (d)

Symptoms at this level include:
Brain
Musculoskeletal
Gastrointestinal
Genitourinary
Dermal

No symptoms at this level

Tissue levels

Pi + Calcium (c)

Bone   Brain   Muscle
Tendon
Ligament
Skin
Gut
Joints

(b) Pi

(a) Pi

Birth

Years

(a) Genetic defect causes phosphate (Pi) retention from birth.
(b) Pi dammed back into bloodstream and along with calcium (Ca^{2+}) is widely distributed to tissues.
(c) Excess accumulation Pi + Ca^{2+} cause malfunction of affected areas.
(d) Joints are finally damaged to cause osteoarthritis.

Figure 2.1

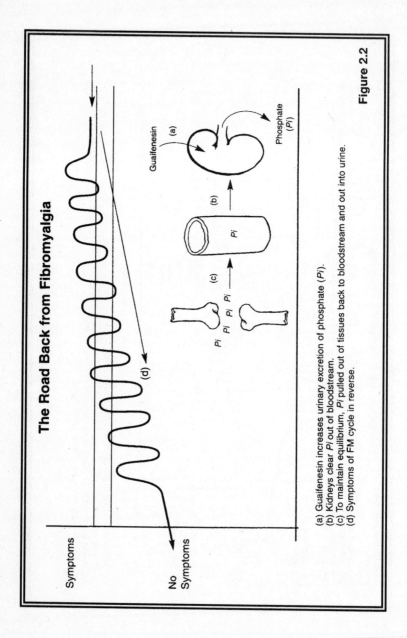

The Road Back from Fibromyalgia

Symptoms

No Symptoms

(a) Guaifenesin increases urinary excretion of phosphate (*Pi*).
(b) Kidneys clear *Pi* out of bloodstream.
(c) To maintain equilibrium, *Pi* pulled out of tissues back to bloodstream and out into urine.
(d) Symptoms of FM cycle in reverse.

Figure 2.2

tion. The first two or three clearing bouts may be quite unpleasant and possibly alarming. Becoming decidedly worse is at least comforting in the promise it holds of better days ahead. We do not believe the bad days are due to the medication's side effects, because no significant side effects have been reported. Instead, they're a tribute to the efficacy of the drug and the speed of reversal.

No one enjoys the initial intensity of reversal—but we did not invent the disease, we merely try to administrate its treatment. If you were born with a low pain threshold, it's not your fault. You'll feel the purging effects more than a higher-threshold person will. We have no soothing words except to say, "Get on with it." Why not get started and get yourself to a better life? One of our favorite patient quotes alluded to the intensity of her cleansing process: "I'm only smiling so that I don't kill you."

Maybe you're asking yourself if you have the strength to endure this onslaught. A related question is: What are the alternatives? To do nothing is to get worse. The disease progresses no matter what you've been told. This is blatantly obvious to fibromyalgics, if not always to the doctors who treat them. Isn't it a fact that you've already tried too many medications, herbs, and adjustments? There was probably an initial relief afforded by these, and by the antidepressant, pain, and sedative medications. As you've developed more symptoms, doctors have progressively added more to the pile. Accepting patchwork symptom suppression with chemical quick fixes eventually fails. No one has to tell you that your symptoms simply resurge, strengthen, and ultimately break through any attempt at medicinal masking.

Chapter 3

◆

Hypoglycemia

One afternoon when I was fifteen I came home from school and collapsed on my bed confused and exhausted. I didn't have enough strength to get up; I couldn't think clearly; I hurt all over. Fast-forward several decades. My diagnosis of fibromyalgia includes hypoglycemia. I took the diagnosis of FM very seriously and reordered my life in the ways required to handle the disease. I got better, slowly, but not fully. It wasn't until I committed to handling my hypoglycemia that startling improvement began.

When I ate correctly I didn't have to sleep half of every day; I didn't have such huge battles with recurring depression; I didn't have the druglike craving for food that resulted in obesity. My commitment to the hypoglycemia "diet" was undertaken not because I wanted to lose weight, but that was a happy side effect. Suddenly I had enough energy to move my body. I knew that exercise is a crucial component of a healthy life, but until I started eating correctly I didn't have enough energy to walk across the room, let alone do any kind of exercise. One good thing kept leading to another. Eating well gave me energy to move, and that in turn made it much easier to exercise, which in turn stimulated endorphins (the body's natural pain reliever). Eating well = more energy = less weight = less pain. This happy cycle resulted in the slow loss of sixty pounds that have stayed off.

Testing this hypothesis caused me quite a bit of grief. When I eat poorly my energy level collapses, my pain increases, my brain gets confused, depression returns. There are quite a few things I can't eat, but I don't feel deprived—I feel energized. After five years my body is much move forgiving of the small transgressions that occur, but I won't ever be able to eat in the manner of most of the population, and I don't want to.

—*Gretchen, South Carolina*

Hypoglycemia is a frequent, unwelcome companion to fibromyalgia, and a contributing factor to your lack of energy. As boring as it may be, let's say it again. Determining whether or not you have this additional misery is an important step. The symptoms of these two conditions interweave, and this overlap makes working with them more than a little challenging. And then, of course, you can certainly reverse fibromyalgia while ignoring your blood sugar problems—but don't expect a full energy boost if you do.

Many names slipped into the lexicon before our medical forebears knew what they were seeing or testing. At times they weren't even sure what they were describing. In the case of the term *hypoglycemia,* however, they were right on target. *Hypo* implies too little of something, and *glycemia* refers to sugar in the circulation. Putting the two together works out, appropriately enough, to mean "low blood sugar."

Let's review a little bit of what we discussed in our prologue. Most hypoglycemics have a repetitive set of complaints in common. Oddly enough, we can use those symptoms diagnostically with more accuracy than relying on a bunch of numbers obtained from blood tests. They neatly divide into two distinguishable kinds, but only one cluster is sufficiently unique to confirm the diagnosis. We call these the acute symptoms of hypoglycemia. Their expression is explosive, and their intense nature leaves little doubt that something awful is afoot.

First might appear a feeling of faintness that doesn't often progress to actual passing out (syncope). As blood sugar levels fall, eventual salvation comes from the timely intervention of the hormone adrenaline (epinephrine). Known as the "flight-or-fight hormone," it responds fiercely, and is dramatically successful in its rescue mission. It's adrenaline that saves us from dropping to the floor in a dead faint—but it hits with alarming intensity. That's what induces the following list, the acute symptoms of hypoglycemia:

1. Internal shakiness or actual hand tremors

2. Cool, clammy skin or sweating

3. Forceful or rapid heartbeat

4. Acute anxiety in the pit of the stomach

5. Frontal pressure headache

6. Panic attacks

In whatever combination these symptoms appear, sufficiently abrupt and overwhelming to suggest som chemical rush. They usually strike about three to four hours after eating. The attack is especially forceful if the last meal included caffeine, sugar, and heavy starches such as potatoes, pasta, or rice. They can also occur during the night, when their intensity abruptly awakens the patient with a pounding heart and already in deep fright.

The other cluster of complaints is what we label the chronic symptoms of hypoglycemia. They account for the steady disturbances that last day and night independent of fasting or satiety. Some people experience them all at once; others, only a handful. The problem with the chronic symptoms is that they overlap so many other conditions. Still, combining the two groupings, acute and chronic, should alert even a relatively untrained physician into making the diagnosis.

Hypoglycemia's chronic symptoms include: fatigue, irritability, nervousness, depression, insomnia, apathy, listlessness, facial or chest flushing, impaired memory and concentration, as well as anxiety. The list enlarges as we add blurring of vision, nasal congestion, ringing in the ears, leg or foot cramps, and numbness and tingling of the hands, feet, or parts of the face such as the lips. There is also dizziness expressed as sensations of faintness. Headaches are usually in the frontal area and may be acute or chronic, often felt as if wearing a rubber band around the forehead. The intestinal tract also announces distress with the so-called irritable bowel syndrome. This consists of nausea, gas, bloating, cramps, and periodic constipation alternating with loose stools or diarrhea. Muscle stiffness is quite disturbing and common in some hypoglycemics. As you can see, this list of chronic symptoms clearly overlaps those of fibromyalgia. That's why correcting only one condition still leaves behind a bunch of symptoms.

Does hypoglycemia occur without fibromyalgia? Of course it does. How do you know for certain if you have one or the other, or both? Hands are great diagnostic tools, as we advocated in the prologue. Working them to seek out swollen areas can be reliably used to separate the two illnesses. Though there is a stiffness or tightness in hypoglycemia, there are no palpable lumps and bumps unless the patient suffers from both conditions, a situation we refer to as fibroglycemia.

If you're confused by now, imagine a physician's dilemma when trying to sort out hypoglycemia, fibromyalgia, hypothyroidism, and a host of other chronic energy-depriving illnesses. Patients feel totally miserable. Scheduled appointment minutes with physicians are eaten up by the litany of complaints. It's enough to make doctors turn in their diplomas. Both patient and professional are victims of this complexity crammed into illnesses that have no simple definitions. But bear with us and we'll do our best to explain some of this in simple terms.

WHAT DOES HYPOGLYCEMIA MEAN TO TISSUES?

For years I listened to everybody (parents, teachers, doctors, diet books) tell me to eat the kind of nutritious "meals" we were taught in school. Lots of good carbs, not much bad fat, and be careful with the protein. I could never understand why I not only didn't lose much weight, but felt *awful* most of the time, with little energy, headachy, and sleepy in midday. No one ever understood I was always so lethargic.

—*Phyllis, North Carolina*

Hypoglycemia is best defined as "sugar levels insufficient for satisfying cerebral requirements," what we popularly call brain glucopenia. Unlike other tissues, the brain relies primarily on glucose for fuel. It burns incredible amounts because of its unrelenting level of activity. Since the brain's foremost instinct is survival, a drop in blood sugar levels evokes urgent responses.

The instigator is always a carbohydrate load abetted by a somewhat jerky release of insulin. In a normal person, insulin thrusts that might excessively drop sugar levels are readily thwarted by well-disciplined, counterregulatory hormones. The sad plight of hypoglycemic patients is that insulin control and the regulatory safety nets simultaneously malfunction. The result is a systemwide disaster.

What exactly are carbohydrates and why are they so daunting to a person with hypoglycemia? Simply put, carbohydrates are composed of carbon, hydrogen, and oxygen. Because of their particular alignment, they're more easily converted to glucose than are other fuel sources. Table sugar (sucrose) or sugars from fruit (fructose), honey (maltose), and milk (lactose) are known as simple carbohydrates. Starches such as bread, pasta, rice, potatoes, cereals, peas, and beans are structured differently and are known as complex carbohydrates. Like other digestible carbohydrates, they're ultimately converted to glucose during the processing needed for intestinal absorption. They're then either immediately consumed for energy or soon distributed all over the body for storage. They become part of the energy reserves warehoused particularly by the liver.

At this point we should pause and pay a visit to a million or so tiny islands located in the pancreas, named islets of Langerhans for their discoverer. Those clusters nurture highly specialized cells with specified duties for both the production and storage of the hormone insulin. Within five to ten minutes after you start to eat carbohydrates, glucose courses through your bloodstream and assails the portals of these pancreatic beta cells, demanding the release of insulin.

Insulin eagerly spurts into the bloodstream for distribution to the many tissues it affects. Like all messengers, its unique structure has reserved spaces in private receptors on the outer surface of cell membranes. Other hormones are not allowed to enter insulin's designated parking areas. For our purposes, we need only dwell on the effect insulin has on muscles, fat cells, and the liver. Given the sheer mass of our bulging muscles, they're the structures most heavily targeted by insulin.

There are deciphering stations locked within recesses of each cell's many insulin receptors. There, instructions are interpreted for the tiers of second and third messengers that lie waiting like so many pony-express riders to relay the incoming mail. Insulin is the same substance no matter where it docks, but the translators in different tissues speak only in their native chemical tongues. That's the amazing thing about hormones: They announce what they want done but have different chores for different tissues. That's why fat (adipocyte), muscle (myocyte), and liver (hepatocyte) cells are each permitted their own method for carrying out insulin's dictates.

Insulin is released into a vein that first bathes the liver. That organ always gets the first read of the freshly imprinted message. It usually extracts much of the glucose for its own requirements, but never all of it. It converts excess sugar into glycogen, the storage form of glucose. A large energy pool is thus created within the liver for the future needs of downstream correspondents. As a result, there's always a readily available source to satisfy other organs and structures. The liver will obligingly release a bit at a time upon request from hungry places all over the body. The brain is a privileged first-dibs recipient of this supply-upon-demand because it works considerably harder than the other tissues. When you're the boss, you get your way, and the brain prefers glucose.

The liver's position in the abdomen is such that it obtains what's called first-pass choices for all newly absorbed nutrients. Besides glucose, insulin urges the liver to take up as many amino and fatty acids as it can handle. For this reason, each meal is a feast as far as the liver is concerned. Everything it extracts is either stored or repackaged for exportation. Whatever it ignores at first glance is allowed to escape downstream to the omnivorous muscles and fat cells.

Once beyond the liver, insulin spreads out to service other tissues. Fat cells, true to their name, always interpret the message as a call to snatch up the fatty acids drifting by. They don't challenge instructions even when they're already overladen and bulging. They only focus on what insulin tells them to do. On top of that, fat cells are gluttons and don't much care what type of fat is being delivered. Their preassigned duty is to warehouse for whatever the future might hold. Once absorbed, the body never wastes food. What is not immediately transformed into energy or inserted to form structures will be saved and guarded with all the fat cell's primal might.

Muscle cells do physiologic handstands when insulin connects up with them. They're not picky, and they never lack appetite. When insulin appears, cell doors are flung wide open to allow glucose to enter, and it doesn't stop there. Insulin enlists cohorts deep inside the cell, getting them to read the fine print in its message. In response, muscles dispatch glucose down a chemical chain for distribution to specific sites. Glucose is then either metabolized into ATP energy or tagged for storage in limited amounts as muscle glycogen.

SO WHAT GOES WRONG?

> Before I started the hypoglycemic diet, I was just getting sicker and sicker. My blood sugars were on the rise, and I was scared to death of diabetes. I've been conscious of good nutrition all my adult life and have tried to eat sensibly. Unfortunately, I had bought the party line that seems to be rampant in this country, and my diet was full of complex carbohydrates—whole-grain breads, legumes, et cetera. Every morning I would eat a big bowl of cooked oat bran. By the time I was finished, I could barely get out of the chair.
>
> —*Cris, Sault Ste. Marie, Michigan*

What causes the precipitous drop in blood sugar we described above—the drop that scares the brain into ordering the release of a flurry of hormones? We've seen how effectively our bodies work to clear glucose out of the bloodstream when we eat carbohydrates. We've seen how efficiently our bodies store the excess fuel we eat as food. The whole system is set up so that nothing goes to waste. What, then, goes wrong?

We eat our meal mixtures, and glucose sooner or later appears in the bloodstream. It was once thought that the walls of blood vessels didn't pay too much attention to glucose circulating through. They were thought to be mainly conduits that channeled gases, building materials, and nutrients from place to place. Now we know that blood vessels are like little spies that use a few strategically placed sensors within their lining to send signals to the brain concerning sugar concentration.

Hypoglycemia fits well into our everyday jargon because most people know the term and what it means. Yet, as you can interpret from the above paragraph, it's a bit imprecise because it only describes the situation in the bloodstream. To remedy this misnomer, we use *glucopenia* in medical jargon as a more descriptive word to denote sugar deprivation. When we tag it onto any parts of the body we're discussing, it identifies the problem at that particular site. Thus, the real problem in hypoglycemia is *brain glucopenia*. It's the brain, not any other part of the body, that sets the comedy of errors that is hypoglycemia in motion.

With current technology, it should be easy to set a numerical definition for normal and low blood sugar, just as we do with cholesterol and liver enzymes. Unfortunately, it isn't that simple. A time-honored number has been fifty milligrams per deciliter of blood (50 mg./dl.) as the number below which hypoglycemia is said to exist. The problem is that this number doesn't reflect what patients actually feel. Many people drop well below this number and suffer no symptoms. Others react with full-blown hypoglycemia although their tests reveal only so-called normal blood sugar readings. What we've learned from this is that in each brain there is a set number, an individually programmed number that sets off an alarm. To put it simply: When your blood sugar falls below your brain's magic number, your brain panics.

Given these facts, what good is the standard five-hour glucose tolerance test often used to diagnose hypoglycemia? The answer is that, in our opinion, it's no good. It's grueling and the results befuddling since we can't rely on any given number for diagnosis. And even if we could, we're gambling that a blood specimen would be extracted at the precise moment the blood sugar drops, not one minute before nor after. With these facts in mind, it's clear that there had better be a better method for diagnosing hypoglycemia than this blood test.

The solution is radical in its simplicity, and endearingly old-fashioned all at once. We just need to listen to what patients have to say. How do you *feel* when you eat sugar or heavy starches? After thousands of cases, we've come to believe that patient-given clues are all we really need to make the diagnosis.

Now that we've identified the brain as the culprit, what actually happens to cause your symptoms? The brain whips up frenetic responses when it senses serious peril to its own survival. Unlike other tissues, it depends almost exclusively on glucose for its unrestricted functions, so when your blood sugar falls below the brain's magic number it metabolically screams for dear life. And those screams are the acute symptoms. Keep this scenario in the back of your mind, because we'll touch on it again in the next section.

HOW DOES HYPOGLYCEMIA AFFECT ENERGY PRODUCTION?

> No one could figure out why a five-year-old would continually faint. But I did. Controlling the hypoglycemia solved the problem . . . forty years later!
>
> —*Morgan M., New York*

What does this extended dialogue have to do with feeling listless? After all, this book is about the lack of energy, not about panic attacks. Bear with us, because we're closing in on the problem.

As we have seen, the brain is well warned of any possible disruption of its energy supply, and an alarm goes off as blood glucose levels decrease. There are two basic reasons why blood sugar goes into free fall. It can be caused by an excessive release of insulin, the same reaction experienced by a diabetic who has accidentally taken too large a dose. Or the body can for some reason experience a delayed or inadequate release of what are known as the counterregulatory hormones. These are the body's natural way of putting the brakes on insulin. First the brain orders the pituitary to release growth hormone, and when this fails to work quickly enough a command is sent to the adrenal gland to release cortisol. But cortisol is also a slow responder, so the pancreas is directed to release glucagon, which also needs time to do its job.

When, despite the above hormones, the blood sugar continues to fall, the brain really goes into a tizzy. The adrenal gland maintains a second hormone, adrenaline, at the ready for countering excessive insulin onslaughts on blood sugar. Instant nerve signals from the brain are all that's needed to evoke a response that will block insulin effects within one to two minutes. But the brain doesn't gamble on just one (albeit powerful) protector. When it's frightened, it regularly arouses its entire defensive nerve and hormonal militia.

A single episode of hypoglycemia leaves the brain a bit befuddled. Frequent, repetitive bouts quickly dull the brain's perception of its own glucopenia. Each successive carbohydrate feast evokes a progressively less forceful counterattacking response. It's as though the brain becomes drugged and dormant. Repeated attacks also promote partial deafness of the salvage systems. Adrenaline sits complacently in its adrenal corner, refusing to come out for the next round. Deprived of its best fighter, the body must now be saved by the slower-acting hormones. Yet their level of response is also blunted by repeated rounds of carbohydrate-induced hypo-glycemia.

All these tasks drain the body's energy and then whittle away and eventually deplete energy stores. As we know, the brain is a huge consumer, and the involvement of all the assorted glands both in manufacturing and releasing hormones is even more draining. It's no wonder that hypoglycemics are tired!

THE HYPOGLYCEMIA DIET

> I started on the liberal diet Dr. St. Amand recommends for hypoglycemia, and I feel better than I have for years. I am a forty-four-year-old black man with no predisposi-tion to diabetes. I have suffered with low blood sugar symptoms for ten years and was recently diagnosed with panic disorder syndrome. I was given 20 mg. of Celexa daily. Until reading Dr. St. Amand's article I had no idea that high-intensity carbohydrate intolerance was the cul-prit for many of my symptoms, including inner shaking, heart palpitations, and severe anxiety. Since the new diet I have stopped taking Celexa with no problems.
>
> —*I. F., California*

Some of you would have been just as happy beginning the chapter here. Fortunately, you don't have to grasp everything we've written in order to get your energy back. The solution is a lot simpler than the problem is: You just have to follow a few simple dietary measures.

Many persuasive arguments can be made for the fact that our modern diet is not what we were designed to eat. That may be why caffeine and carbohydrates are such potent villains. Sorry, hypoglycemics, there is no getting around this even though it's not what you want to hear: You *must* avoid the interdicted foods and maintain dietary restrictions long enough to get well. Beyond exposing the cause and providing the solution, we can't do more than steer you to the task at hand. Lacking a magic pill, you're left to cope by yourself. Although abstinence is difficult, the body will quickly reward you with the sweetness of energy. Achieve this much and you'll repair another defective spoke of your ruptured energy wheel.

We hinted at the necessary corrective steps when we described the series of events that follow insulin surges. Only carbohydrates create a huge demand for its release. We've come to the bottom line now. It's time emphatically to state that *you absolutely must adhere to the dietary restrictions we spell out below if you want to get well.*

When we reach the point of explaining the corrective measures to our patients, we routinely brace ourselves for the forthcoming shaking of heads, complaints, and heavy sighs. Our pat response is, "We don't invent diseases; we only administrate them." Our job is to warn of pitfalls and outline what foods must be avoided. We deeply regret taking away so many comfort foods and tasty treats, but we can neither bargain away necessary restrictions nor dispense self-discipline. By the time you're an out-and-out hypoglycemic, you've already raided your energy bank and dried up the account. *Like every other illness we talk about in this book, if you've developed the symptoms, you're broke!* You can no longer write checks until you've reestablished a positive balance.

Cheating is a guarantee of self-defeat. There are no effective shortcuts like chromium picolinate or other dietary supplements—no matter what the advertisements say. You can sometimes get by if you try eating small meals all day long. Eventually, however, you have to sleep, and when you do, you'll wake with your body in an uproar.

Taming insulin releases helps nonhypoglycemic fibromyalgics as well. A prime function of insulin is to drive glucose molecules into cells, but it must also tag them with companion phosphates. Once attached, they prevent glucose from escaping back out of the cell. This chemical ritual facilitates storage and assures energy availability for rapid deployment. Obviously, this piggybacking entry of phosphate isn't the greatest thing for the fibromyalgic cell, because it already has trouble extruding excessive phosphate. This is the main reason that the insulin-glucose tandem often further depletes energy production and worsens the fibromyalgia situation.

Insulin also signals certain kidney cells to reabsorb some of the previously filtered serum phosphate that was destined for elimination. These salvaged ions are then returned to the bloodstream and widely distributed to various tissues throughout the body. Cells most severely affected by hypoglycemia and fibromyalgia—muscle and brain—are the very ones most compliant with insulin's demands. Those hyperresponsive structures heed commands and absorb the largest amounts of phosphate. It follows that curtailing carbohydrate intake diminishes intracellular phosphate, and that's the very thing we need in fibromyalgia.

For these reasons, fibromyalgics, not only the carbohydrate-craving ones, may enjoy some symptomatic improvement by avoiding sugars and heavy starches. Let's face it, there's lag time and much cycling ahead before guaifenesin gradually reverses fibromyalgia. In the meantime, highly encouraging energy gains and symptomatic abatement may come from this type of dieting. Some quick rewards include easing the fibrofog and drowsiness that follow a carbohydrate meal. Morning fatigue may be lessened simply by avoiding the heavier carbohydrates before bed. Irritable bowel syndrome almost always improves significantly in a few days. For nonhypoglycemic fibromyalgics, three weeks on the restricted diet is plenty of time to experience its benefits. The flip side is that if nothing improves, there's no need to stay on it. So often are our words misinterpreted that we repeat: *Though it may prove energizing, there is no required diet for fibromyalgia.*

Perfectly followed, the diet will begin providing increased energy within ten days. Hypoglycemic patients are at least 75 percent improved within one month; within two, totally cleared. If they haven't cheated during that time, they should have regained whatever reserves their individual metabolism permits. Let's accept that most of you with hypoglycemia may always have more limited resources than others. We each have assets and capacities. Some of us are taller, prettier, brighter, more innovative, stronger, and faster. Some carry genes for diabetes, some for cancer, and some for heart disease. This is the stuff of real life. But that shouldn't stop all of us from achieving our own personal best.

After the first two months, you may begin eating foods that are least likely to cause problems. The safest are those with a low *glycemic index,* a term defined as "the least demanding of insulin responses." Potatoes, pasta, and sucrose are high on the index charts and may always have to be limited according to the degree of your problem. Brown and wild rice are safer initial forays than a glob of the white variety. Experiment with small servings at first. Suffering no adverse effects indicates that you can handle a particular food. Then you have to learn how often your metabolism will permit you to cheat. It will take you several trial-and-error splurges before you become confident about what you can eat, how much, and how often.

Venture carefully into this process. Don't go too far or too fast. Remember that you've been good for a couple of months and rebuilt your reserve account. Even infrequent "cheats" are checks written against your balance, and you must be able to cover them metabolically. Your symptoms *will* return if you don't practice self-discipline. Sneak up on the diet and cheat only with your body's permission. Back off immediately at the first signs of trouble. Excessive dietary indiscretions usually evoke the acute symptoms of hypoglycemia within three to three and a half hours. If you blow it, begin all over again, counting forward from the time of the last cheat. Resume the diet for a few more weeks until you feel perfectly well. On your next attempt, cheat less frequently and go easier on the forbidden foods. It's been said that we learn best by our failures.

It may take you a year of hunting and pecking to finalize your diet. In the process, you'll observe for yourself how much stress, injury, or illness drain energy. When you eat your way into adverse moments while trying to establish your final diet, don't ignore a lesson learned. You can avoid trouble by minimizing your carbohydrate intake ahead of time. Once you get used to doing without caffeine, you may never choose to go back to it for a very simple reason: It demands too much expenditure from your energy account and provides very little reward. The same applies to risky foods that you find easy to avoid. Save your cheats for things you really, really like.

Mercifully, in our experience, most hypoglycemics lose their cravings after about ten days. However, we can't duck one issue. The first few days can be quite difficult, and patients may suffer from increased fatigue and other carbohydrate-withdrawal symptoms. Though the situation gradually improves after the first two weeks, obese patients may have more difficulty and experience unrelenting cravings. One patient said it well: "I've never met a carbohydrate I didn't like." We'll delve deeper into reasons for this in chapter 5, on obesity.

Friends will tempt you when you dine in their homes or join them in restaurants. You've already heard it too many times: "One little bite won't hurt you." To this there is only one honest retort, "Yes it will!" Other problems sneak in when eating out. Don't hesitate asking if salad dressings and soups contain sugar or starchy thickening agents. Make sure your server understands that you'll get sick if you eat the wrong thing. Insist on confirmation that coffee in the orange-topped carafe is definitely caffeine-free. Some waiters feel no compunction about pouring the real thing to replace the unleaded variety you ordered: They may have run out for the moment and wouldn't dream of making you wait for the new brew. You may not taste the difference, but a few hours later your adrenaline rush will leave you wishing that you could have.

Now, I know this can be a difficult diet for someone to start, but for me it was going to be a rough road—you see, I am a vegetarian. I never in my wildest dreams thought I could give up bread, pastas, rice, fruit, et cetera, as that was my main nourishment. And heaven forbid I would give up sugars! I have FM and I needed my two pots of coffee a day to survive (I thought) but I have given that up also. And guess what? I feel so much better without all that junk (did I call it junk?). I used to *love* it. I incorporate soy and protein drinks in my diet for proteins instead of meat. By the way, I did this cold turkey; for me that was the best way—to jump into the diet with both feet. It is now April 2002, and I plan to live this way forever. My husband joined me in this way of life a year ago and he too plans to stay low carb. By the way, I have lost twenty-six pounds and have never gained it back. I eat a liberal diet now to maintain. I also have low cholesterol. HG eating is a wonderful way to live.

—*Tracy S. (started guai on January 9, 1992;*
HG diet since July 1999)

The Basic Hypoglycemia Diet

(The ensuing diet is designed for control of hypoglycemia. Those hypoglycemics who need to lose weight should refer to chapter 5. Once weight loss has been accomplished, the following diet will preserve it. Underweight hypoglycemics should eat added servings of the sugar-free bread, dairy products, fruits, and grains we list below. Otherwise they might lose too much weight.)

MEATS   All meats, fish, shellfish, and fowl are allowed, except cold cuts that contain sugar. Check labels carefully. Low-fat and nonfat cold cuts usually have added dextrose or corn syrup. Bacon and ham are acceptable although they do list sugar on the labels. It cooks off and isn't a problem. Heavily coated hams should be washed free of their sweet coating. Meats are allowed in unlimited quantity.

DAIRY PRODUCTS   Milk (nonfat, whole, low fat), cream (heavy and sour), unsweetened yogurt, as well as natural cheeses (no processed cheese in foods, in bulk, or sliced). This includes cottage and ricotta cheeses, and goat cheese. Butter, margarine, and eggs (or egg substitutes) are all allowed in unlimited quantities.

FRUITS Limit: 1 piece of fruit every 4 hours. *No fruits except the ones listed,* and don't drink fruit juice, except 1 cup of unsweetened orange, grapefruit, or tomato.

Apples
Apricots
Blackberries (½-cup limit)
Blueberries (½-cup limit)
Boysenberries
Cantaloupe
Casaba melon (1-wedge limit)
Coconut (fresh)
Grapefruit
Honeydew melon
    (1-wedge limit)
Lemons (juice for seasoning)
Limes (juice for seasoning)
Nectarines
Oranges
Papaya
Peaches
Pears
Plums
Raspberries
Strawberries
Tangerines
Tomato juice
V8 Juice

VEGETABLES
Artichokes
Asparagus
Avocados
Bean sprouts
Beets
Broccoli
Brussels sprouts
Cabbage (limit 1 cup per day)
Carrots
Cauliflower
Celery
Celery root
Chard
Chicory
Chinese cabbage
    (limit 2 cups per day)
Chives
Cucumber
Daikon (long, white radish)
Eggplant

Endive
Escarole
Garlic
Greens (mustard, beet)
Jicama
Kale
Leeks
Lettuce
Mushrooms
Okra
Olives
Onions
Parsley
Peas
Peppers
   (red, green, yellow, etc.)
Pickles
   (dill, sour; limit 1 per day)
Pimiento
Pumpkin

Radicchio
Radish
Rhubarb
Salad greens
Sauerkraut
Scallions (green onions)
Snow peas
Spinach
String beans (green or yellow)
Summer squash
   (crookneck yellow or green)
Tomatoes
Turnips
Vegetable sprouts
Water chestnuts
Watercress
Winter squash
   (acorn, butternut,
   buttercup, spaghetti, etc.)
Zucchini

NUTS

Almonds
Brazil
Butternuts
Cashews
Filberts
Hazelnuts
Hickory nuts
Macadamia nuts

Peanuts
Pecans
Pignoli (pine nuts)
Pistachios
Soy nuts
Sunflower seeds
Walnuts

BREADS Limit: 3 total slices of sugar-free white, whole wheat, sourdough, light rye, corn tortilla *or* sugar-free flatbread, pita, or puffed rice cakes per day. Use no more than 2 slices at one time.

DESSERTS
Sugar-free Jell-O
Custard (made with cream and artificial sweetener)
Cheesecake (nut-crusted or without crust, made with cream cheese, sour cream, and artificial sweeteners)

BEVERAGES
Artificially sweetened drink mixes like Crystal Light, Country Time, etc.
Club soda, zero-carbohydrate flavored soda waters
Decaffeinated coffee
Sodas with no sugar or caffeine
Weak or decaffeinated tea
Bourbon, cognac, gin, rum, Scotch, vodka, dry wine *(after 2 months on a perfect diet, most hypoglycemics can tolerate 1 drink only, occasionally more)*

CONDIMENTS AND SPICES
All spices including seeds (fresh or dried)
All imitation flavorings
Horseradish
Sugar-free sauces such as hollandaise, mayonnaise, mustard, ketchup, soy sauce, Worcestershire sauce
Sugar-free salad dressings
Oil and vinegar (all types)

MISCELLANEOUS

Atkins bars, shakes, baking mixes (and other low-carbohydrate brands)
All fats
Carob powder
Caviar
Flour (gluten, soy, or nut only)
Gravy made with gluten or soy flour only
Tofu
Popcorn (1 cup popped)
Pork rinds
Wheat germ
Puffed rice, shredded wheat, or other sugar-free cereals
2 tacos or 2 enchiladas (2 corn tortillas at one time only)
Wondercocoa
Xanthan gum

If cholesterol is a problem, avoid cold cuts except sugar-free turkey. Trim all visible fat off meat. Remove the skin from poultry. Broil or grill foods instead of frying. Avoid any but low-fat cheese, as well as heavy cream, solid margarine, hollandaise sauce, and macadamia nuts. Replace whole eggs with egg whites or Egg Beaters. Use liquid margarine only. Nuts should be dry-roasted and not oil-coated. Use canola or olive oil.

For eighteen months I lay awake every night between 3 and 4 A.M. with what I could only describe as panic attacks. However, after I had completed my divorce and was feeling better emotionally than any time in my life— I had nothing to panic about. I finally figured out that my adrenaline surges had little to do with my emotions and everything to do with what I was eating—a high-carbohydrate diet. I switched to low-carb eating and the "panic" attacks vanished. In the end, I'm thankful for hypoglycemia because it's what led me to guaifenesin as a treatment for fibromyalgia.

—*Roberta, Bellingham, Washington*

Perhaps you still have questions regarding the diet. Most of those we're asked arise from confusion concerning the nature of carbohydrates. Many people have difficulty understanding why they can't have a few bites of potato instead of the three slices of sugar-free bread in their daily allotment. They're more accustomed to diets in which calories are simply totaled, and kept under a certain number. These diets cumulate the total number of calories from meat, fruit, vegetables, sweets, and liquids. If the total is sufficiently low, weight loss should begin without regard to the dietary mix. Based on this, carbohydrate substitution, gram for gram, seems logical. Unfortunately, this type of math doesn't work for our purposes, because carbohydrates are not all the same. The amount of insulin stimulated by each variety is quite different. This has been measured, and a scale produced called the glycemic index. Copies of this index are available at your library or bookstore, or on the Internet; there's also a simplified version in our first book. While the hypoglycemic diet doesn't correlate exactly with the glycemic index, and certain questions have been raised about its absolute accuracy, it does provide a sort of framework for those who are interested in the concept.

I still have my bad days, and as I told Claudia to write on my chart, *"It's the food, stupid!!"* (and it is).

—*Marty Ross, California*

Presently, hypoglycemics are gaining resources thanks to the popularity of the Dr. Robert Atkins diets, *Protein Power*, *The Zone*, and *The Carbohydrate Addict* programs. But when using low-carbohydrate diets other than ours, remain vigilant. Some of those diets are primarily designed for weight loss and not for control of hypoglycemia. Especially be aware that they may include caffeine as an ingredient—for example, in coffee and chocolate. Check the labels on wrappers and packages. Be sure nothing slips by you that might destroy what benefits you've accrued from your prolonged dietary efforts. In addition, it's important when reading labels to match serving sizes to the posted carbohydrate count. Some low-carbohydrate products designed for diabetics do something even trickier by not listing some sweeteners that presumably don't have a huge effect on blood sugar.

In the next chapter are recipes and ideas to start you on your way. Many more are available from Web sites as well as recipe books dedicated to low-carbohydrate dieting. These resources greatly ease the chore of cooking and help you adopt a new way of life. Enjoy your new health and vitality!

Chapter 4

◆

Recipes for Successfully Managing Hypoglycemia

I really don't think of it as a diet anymore. It's just the way I eat. I tell people that if they were sick enough and had gotten the results I got from it, they would too, and they'd be happy to stick to it. I just wish more people could realize the benefits of it. I see so many around me who probably need it, but they think it's too hard and they won't even give it a try.

—*Cris, Sault Ste. Marie, Michigan*

If you're like most people, any mention of the word *diet* is enough to throw you into a panic. For fibromyalgics, this is especially true, because you don't have the energy to make changes. Shopping expeditions can be an ordeal, and thinking up new ways to prepare foods can sound insurmountable. For those who aren't creative in the kitchen, and others who simply find themselves too busy to experiment a bit with our guidelines, the hypoglycemia diet can be daunting. That's why we've included this chapter.

You see, we're all creatures of habit. If you're used to eating the same seven foods and suddenly four of those are eliminated, you'll find yourself eating a diet of the same three foods. Not only does this put you at a nutritional disadvantage, but it gets boring—quickly. If you're hypoglycemic, you're not going to feel better until you change your diet. Even if you only have fibromyalgia, there are some good reasons why this same diet can make you have more energy. Try it—you have nothing to lose but your fatigue!

How I hate my doctors for all those years of feeling sick and nauseous, and always having to have something to eat with me, et cetera, and I hadn't a clue that it was a blood sugar problem. . . . Within days of starting the HG diet I started feeling so much better that my husband became *very* interested in helping me stay on it. I guess I didn't realize how much my mood swings induced by the spiking blood sugar were affecting him. At my age (I'm almost sixty-one) I do not care if I have to eat horse apples. If it makes me feel better, I will do it. I lost weight and felt so much better, and so did my husband. He recently had his cholesterol checked and guess what? All his cholesterol numbers were *better* than ever even though he's eating butter, heavy cream, eggs, et cetera. Amazing! All he did was cut out carbohydrates and Cokes, cookies, sweets, et cetera.

—*Ursula, Albuquerque, New Mexico*

We've done our best to put a variety of dishes in this chapter. Hopefully, after you try a few, you'll get the idea and be able to come up with concoctions of your own. We also have a section about converting recipes to help you, although many of the ones you have now might be just fine.

BEFORE YOU START *(YOU HAVE TO GO TO THE MARKET)*

It's a good idea to stock up on food you can eat. The worst thing on any diet is when you're hungry and you go into the kitchen and start looking and you feel like there's nothing you can eat. I make a couple of big containers of sugar-free Jell-O every weekend so at least I can grab a bowl of that with whipped cream. Slices of cheese and cold cuts are good, too. It's not a bad idea if you can get organized enough to put snack-size or small portions of things in the freezer so you just microwave them and have something to eat in a minute or two.

—*Lou M., Los Angeles, California*

The first thing you have to do is to think about what you *can* eat, and what you'll need for recipes and snacks. Here are some ideas of what you should have on hand. The first time you go to the market to stock your kitchen, make sure you have a copy of your diet with you, and that you know all the ingredients to strictly avoid. Allow plenty of time, because you're going to have to read the labels on practically everything you pick up, especially on packaged and processed foods; these are the easiest places to slip up.

What follows is a list of basic things that it's convenient to have on hand for your new diet. You don't have to buy everything all at once; you can buy things as you'll need them, and maybe get a little extra to keep on hand. This way, you'll always have something to eat in the house. Buy from this list, but do adapt it to what you like. If you don't like barbecue sauce or certain spices, pick something you like instead. Just remember to check the ingredients on anything processed or prepared for hidden sugars.

- Spices are important because without sugar, you'll want something to season your food, and to make dressings and dips: mustard, curry, dill, garlic, ginger, chilies, basil, rosemary, thyme, and so forth. You can use fresh or dried (1 teaspoon of dried herbs is equal to 1 tablespoon of fresh). Don't buy the jumbo sizes of dried spices; they do lose flavor over time, especially if they're in bottles. Use horseradish if you like the taste—either bottled or fresh, which needs to be grated. (Add to cream or sour cream for a sauce, or to cream cheese to roll inside slices of meat for a snack.) If you like spicy food, you can use dried, canned, or fresh chilies, or hot pepper sauces without sugar. You'll have to check the labels carefully.
- Oils for cooking and dressings—all flavors are acceptable. If you buy smallish bottles on sale, you can add your own spices to them and use while cooking or to season cooked vegetables. A few cloves of garlic in a squeeze bottle full of olive oil near the stove can really make preparing vegetables easy and delicious. Make sure you have vinegar as well. There are many herbed ones, and all vinegars are acceptable.
- Liquid Smoke—a very small drop adds a lot of flavor.
- Sugar-free soy sauce—it's out there, just check the labels.

- Sweet pepper spread, garlic, pesto, and olive pastes (usually sugar-free, but check them) to add to soups, sauces, mayonnaise, cream, or sour cream for dips. Green peppercorns, capers, olives—keep a few bottles on hand. These can be added to sauces, dips, and salads. Also, artichoke hearts (frozen, bottled, or canned) come in handy.
- Sugar-free syrups—sweetened with Splenda, they have no aftertaste. Fruit flavors for shakes, caramel for desserts, and so on. These can also be added to coffee or tea. (Several brands are Da Vinci, Torani, Carbolyte, and Atkins.)
- Sugar-free maple syrup made with Splenda. Use for low-carbohydrate pancakes, crepes, oatmeal, and so on. It can also be used to flavor vegetables (like squash or carrots) or meats such as ham in place of honey or other sugars.
- Bread crumbs made from sugar-free bread, or from pork rinds—crush for breading, use for dips or nachos. You can also buy these already prepared from Web sites.
- Protein powders—whey, milk, egg, and soy protein powders in various flavors. Use to make protein drinks, as thickeners or breading, and sometimes in baking.
- Low-carb baking mix—there are lots of these now. You can make bread or pancakes with zero carbohydrates. Atkins and Carbolyte are best; there's also Soy Quick baking mix. Atkins and other Web sites now have bread machine mixes that can be used as pizza crust.
- Gelatin packets—keep a store on hand to make puddings and the like.
- Unsweetened coconut and cans of coconut milk—you can buy this grated in bags, a very handy ingredient for curries, desserts, and snacks. You can also cook shrimp or chicken in the milk. Look in health food stores if you can't find these in the regular market.

- Nuts—always keep large bags of nuts. You can crush them and add them to many things, use them as toppings or snacks, and more.
- Sugar-free mayonnaise (or make your own).
- Sugar-free catsup (or make your own).
- Sugar-free barbecue sauce (or make your own). (Note: Sugar-free condiments and preserves can also be purchased from the Web sites listed in the resource section at the back of this book.)
- Chicken, beef, or vegetable stock—there are sugar-free cans in various sizes, or you can buy the cubes. You can use stock as the base for soup, to cook in, for a quick egg-drop soup, or as a snack.
- Sugar-free Jell-O—You can always make a quick snack or dessert.
- Sugar-free puddings—there is a limit on these because of the starch, but especially the five-minute instant ones are handy to have around.
- Eggs—although the egg scare has largely passed, you may still be nervous about the cholesterol in eggs. If the newer studies that repudiated this old urban legend don't comfort you, Egg Beaters and other egg substitutes may certainly be used for custards, quiches, et cetera.
- Margarine or butter—there's no reason to avoid butter, but if you prefer margarine, remember that the liquid ones are better for you than the solids.
- Cans of chilies, especially chipotles and green chilies (ortegas) for stuffing.
- Vegetables—if you have a can or two of green beans, you have a salad (we keep one in the fridge) or a quick delicious soup. This is also true of other canned or frozen vegetables

on the diet. It's a good idea to keep bags of frozen vegetables in the freezer. They stay fresh, and you can always whip something up.

- Meats—tuna, sardines, salmon, chicken meat, and Vienna sausages all make quick snacks or salads. You can also freeze leftovers in small packets. Frozen cooked shrimp and crabmeat are good to have stocked. Bacon and ham are also good; you can freeze them in small portions, or buy dehydrated microwave bacon. Salami and pepperoni are handy for snacks and omelets.

- Cheese—keep several types handy. You should always have cream cheese or ricotta, and a dry cheese such as Parmesan, Romano, feta, or the like. If you like blue cheese, have that or Gorgonzola for sauces or to eat plain. Cheddar, Jack, or whatever else you like can be used for snacks, quiches, and so on.

- Sugar-free tomato or pasta sauces—you can always use these.

- Hearts of palm—can dress up a dreary salad.

- Bamboo shoots—another addition to salads or for stir-fry (crunchy).

- Water chestnuts—slice for stir-fries; put in the blender and use as a thickener.

- Fruit-only jellies.

- Sugar-free peanut butter or other nut butters.

- Wasa, Bran-a-crisp, or any sugar-free flatbread or crackers.

- Soy flour, gluten flour—gluten flour has the most neutral flavor.

- Sugar-free cereal such as oatmeal (unsweetened) or shredded wheat (unsweetened).

- Lemon juice (unsweetened)—for times when you may not have fresh lemons on hand, keep a bottle of this handy in the refrigerator.

- Fruit—it doesn't hurt to have a few bags of frozen strawberries or other fruits on hand. Of course you'll want the
  ones without syrup.

We eat meat (broiled, fried, sautéed, or barbecued) and
vegetables, fresh and frozen with cheese, or browned in
butter, or plain. I boil eggs and use them in salads and/or
soups with fresh vegetables. I sprinkle sunflower seeds or
a few slivered almonds into my salads. And then there's
the cheese: I cut strips of it and use it like bread as an accompaniment for the soups. Sour cream and heavy cream
I make into salad dressings with dill or oregano, or whatever spice for flavor. I make meat patties out of hamburger with Italian seasonings, cayenne pepper, and
onion powder (I use just a touch), grated Parmesan
cheese, and an egg: They taste like sausage and I know
exactly what is in them.

—*Ursula, Albuquerque, New Mexico*

BREAKFAST

Breakfast is an easy meal for hypoglycemics, as long as you
have sugar-free bread and cereal on hand. You can have eggs
any style with breakfast meat or cheese, cottage cheese and a
piece of fruit, low-carb pancakes (get one of the low-carb baking or pancake mixes), or a slice or two of French toast (made
with sugar-free bread and sugar-free maple syrup). You can
also have protein shakes, and yogurt (unsweetened—add your
own sweetener) with a serving of fruit. The recipe for egg custard is in the dessert section, but it is also a delicious way to
start the day. Quiches and frittatas are wonderful, and you can

just cut a portion and microwave it. Many companies also make protein bars, and even breakfast bars, if you're the kind to have breakfast on the go.

Basic Omelet

Makes 1 serving.

> 2 eggs
> 1 tablespoon heavy cream or milk
> 1 tablespoon water
> dash of salt
> dash of pepper
> 2 tablespoons butter

Combine the eggs, cream, water, salt, and pepper. Beat lightly. Melt 2 tablespoons of butter in a nonstick pan until it bubbles. Pour the egg mixture into the pan. Cook for about 2 minutes, pulling the edges inward as they set. Liquid eggs will swirl into their place. When omelet is solid but still soft, flip one side inward to make a half circle, cook for a few more minutes, slide from the pan, and serve.

If you aren't good at this (we're not), preheat the broiler before you start. Then, when the omelet is set and the bottom is cooked, slide the frying pan with the omelet in it under the broiler until the top is cooked. Slide onto a plate and flip one side over.

Fines Herbes: Add chopped parsley, 1 tablespoon snipped chives, and 1 tablespoon snipped dill (or actually, whichever herbs you like) to the eggs before you cook them.

Omelet Variations

Make additions when the omelet is ready to fold over. Cook for a few minutes to heat the filling. You can also pass it under the broiler at this point and accomplish the same thing.

Cheese omelet: ½ cup grated cheese.
Denver omelet: onion, green pepper, and ham.
Spanish omelet: sugar-free tomato sauce.
Western omelet: chopped ham, green pepper, onion, and grated cheese.
Avocado and Swiss cheese.
Spinach and ricotta cheese.
Or sausage, bacon, salami, or any vegetable, with or without cheese.

Cheese Pancakes

Makes 4 to 6 pancakes. (Serves 2.)

½ cup whole-milk ricotta or cottage cheese
3 eggs
1½ tablespoons soy flour or soy protein
1½ tablespoons butter (softened in microwave)
1 teaspoon salt

Combine the ingredients in a blender and blend until smooth. Heat a pan or griddle until very hot, and rub with oil. Cook the pancakes.

Eggs Florentine

Serves 4.

1 16-ounce package frozen chopped spinach
1 tablespoon butter
4–6 eggs
½ cup cream
½ cup water
1½ cups grated mild cheese
1 teaspoon dry mustard

Preheat the oven to 350 degrees. Cook the spinach and mix with butter. Place in the bottom of a baking dish, making little circles in it with a spoon. Break the eggs and drop their contents into the little nests you've just made.

Combine the cream, water, cheese, and mustard in a microwave-safe dish and microwave for 30 seconds. Stir and repeat until sauce is smooth. Pour over the eggs and spinach. Bake for 30 minutes.

Strawberry Protein Drink

Makes 1 16-ounce shake.

½ cup milk
2 teaspoons sugar substitute
½ cup strawberries, fresh or frozen
½ cup cold water
½ cup crushed ice

Combine all the ingredients in a blender and blend until frothy. You can substitute any fresh or frozen fruit (1 serving) and/or sugar-free syrup. If you're using a syrup, be sure to omit the sugar substitute.

Cranberry Oatmeal

This dish is not for a weight-loss diet.

For 2 people—can be adjusted as needed.

    2 cups milk
    1 cup quick oats
    ½ cup dried cranberries
    1 medium apple, peeled, cored, and chopped
    ½ teaspoon cinnamon
    1 tablespoon Da Vinci or other sugar-free syrup (gingerbread or
        cinnamon flavored is best)
    Splenda to taste if needed
    1 teaspoon butter or margarine
    ½ cup heavy cream
    dash of cinnamon
    dash of nutmeg

In a medium saucepan, combine the milk, oats, fruits, ½ teaspoon cinnamon, syrup, and Splenda. Bring to a boil over medium heat. Cover the pan and reduce the heat to medium low. Simmer for 3 to 4 minutes until oatmeal is the consistency you like. Stir several times while it is cooking so it doesn't stick to the pan.

Dish into 2 bowls. Place ½ teaspoon of butter in each dish. Stir. Pour cream on top and put a dash of nutmeg and cinnamon on each serving.

Breakfast Frittata

This is a basic frittata recipe. You can make any mixture you like, adding ham, cheese, Italian sausage, pepperoni, and any leftover vegetables. This is one of those dishes you can use leftovers in, and it's delicious. You can also top with sour cream.

Makes 1 serving.

- 1 small onion, chopped (or 2 scallions, chopped, or ½ cup chopped leek for weight-loss diet or if preferred)
- ½ cup zucchini, chopped into thin strips about 3 inches long
- 1 chopped tomato, seeds removed
- 2 strips bacon, crumbled (or ½ cup of any chopped meat, including pepperoni, ham, sausage)
- 4 eggs, beaten until pale and frothy
- ½ cup grated Swiss, Parmesan, Romano, Gruyère, or Jack cheese.
- 2 tablespoons chopped basil or cilantro

Preheat the oven to 350 degrees. In a skillet, heat 1 tablespoon of olive oil and 1 tablespoon of butter (or 2 tablespoons of olive oil) until bubbly. Cook the onion until it is brown, or, if you're using scallions or leeks, until well cooked. Add the zucchini and cook until soft; add the tomatoes and meat near the end because they only need to be heated through. Add the eggs to the skillet and sprinkle with cheese. As you do so, remove the skillet from the heat. Some people place the skillet in the oven and let it bake. We prefer at this point to pour the mixture into a glass (square or rectangle) baking dish. Put it in the oven and bake for 10 minutes, until firm and fluffy.

Remove from oven. Cut in squares and serve hot or cold. A slice makes a nice breakfast, eaten hot or cold.

Faux Eggs Benedict

Note: This dish is not for a weight-loss diet.

Serves 2.

> 4 eggs
> 4 pieces Canadian bacon
> 2 slices sourdough toast (no sugar)
> ⅓ cup butter
> 2 egg yolks
> 2 teaspoons lemon juice
> dash of cayenne pepper and salt

Poach the eggs, and fry the Canadian bacon until hot. Cut each slice of sourdough toast in half, and top each half with a slice of Canadian bacon and a poached egg. Melt the butter in the microwave until liquid. Put the egg yolks in a bowl or blender. Beat until frothy. Add the lemon juice, salt, and cayenne and continue beating. Very slowly and carefully add the liquid butter and blend until thick. Top the poached eggs with spoonfuls of sauce.

LUNCH

My main symptom has always been severe fatigue. When I experience this fatigue I crave carbohydrates even more. I had a dreadful time trying to stick to the diet, but I kept persisting. I'd make mistakes. I was finally able to do the diet successfully. The results were amazing. I was able to go to the gym and start exercising! I haven't been able to do this in the twenty-plus years I have been dealing with this chronic illness. I am still amazed. I guess it just goes to show that perseverance pays off with the guai protocol and with the HG diet. The lesson to be learned: Don't give up! The protocol works if you work it.

—*Denise B., Syracuse, New York*

For lunch, you'll again find that you have many choices. Salads, as long as you don't use dressings with sugar or croutons made from regular bread, are easy choices. You can make endless combinations: chef's, Caesar, chopped, Greek, Italian, and so on. Egg, salmon, crab, shrimp, and other salads can be made with meat. Even on the weight-loss diet, you can have sandwiches using big lettuce leaves or cabbage leaves as bread, or, on the liberal diet, use a slice of sugar-free bread. You can also make roll-ups with deli meat filled with soft cheese, and chopped pickle or horseradish. Quiches will last for a few days, and you can always eat leftover meat with a salad or soup on the side. Hamburgers, cheeseburgers, and bacon-avocado burgers can be eaten without the bread.

Chef's Salad

Serves 2 as an appetizer, 1 as a main course.

    1½ cups torn romaine lettuce
    ½ cup sliced chicken or turkey
    ½ cup sliced ham
    ¼ cup sliced cheese such as Cheddar or Swiss
    2 hard-boiled eggs, cut in half
    Other salad ingredients such as olives, radishes, or cucumbers
        for garnish

Place the lettuce in a bowl and arrange the other ingredients on the top. Top with your favorite sugar-free dressing.

Chicken Caesar Salad

Makes 1 serving.

1 grilled chicken breast (or serving of shrimp or blackened fish)
½ tablespoon olive oil if grilling or broiling, or 1 tablespoon if
    pan-frying
romaine lettuce or romaine mixture
sliced cherry tomatoes, if desired
croutons made from sugar-free bread or pork rinds

John Oldrate's Caesar Dressing:
1 egg (or equal amount egg substitute)
1 tablespoon lemon juice
1 garlic clove, chopped fine
1 teaspoon dry mustard or Dijon mustard
1 teaspoon Worcestershire sauce
dash of Tabasco sauce
salt and pepper
2 chopped anchovies, drained and mashed (if desired), or a
    squeeze of anchovy paste from tube
½ cup olive oil
½ cup grated Parmesan cheese

Brush the chicken with olive oil mixed with lemon juice. Salt and pepper the chicken, and grill, broil, or pan-fry.

To make the dressing, drop the egg (in the shell) into boiling water for 30 seconds. Crack the egg into a wooden bowl. (This is done to avoid the risk from using a raw egg. If you're still nervous, use one of the egg substitutes.) Add the lemon, garlic, mustard, Worcestershire sauce, Tabasco, salt and pepper, and anchovies if you are using them. Whisk until well beaten, then add the oil, slowly whisking as you go. Lastly, add the cheese.

Arrange the romaine in a bowl with the cherry tomatoes, if using, and the croutons. (For a liberal diet, you can use ½ cup sourdough croutons. For a strict diet, use pork rind croutons.) Pour on the dressing and toss. Sprinkle more Parmesan over the top and serve.

Greek Salad

Serves 2.

> 3 cups chopped lettuce
> 1 large tomato, cut into bite-size pieces
> 1 large cucumber, cut into bite-size pieces
> 1 large green pepper, chopped
> ½ cup olive oil
> 2 teaspoons red wine vinegar
> 1 teaspoon lemon juice
> ½ cup crumbled feta cheese
> salt and pepper
> 1 tablespoon chopped fresh oregano or 1 teaspoon dried
> 1 teaspoon chopped parsley or basil (you could even use dill)
> 10 chopped kalamata olives
> 1 large scallion, chopped

Combine the ingredients in a salad bowl and toss. If you're not on the weight-loss diet, you can add 1 chopped red onion, if desired.

Egg Salad Variations

Chop the desired number of hard-boiled eggs with a fork until fine. Add sugar-free mayonnaise to the desired consistency. (Some people like theirs dry, while others like it gooey.) For variations, try adding any of the following to taste:

Dill
Curry powder and cilantro
Mustard, dry or Dijon
Cumin

Spoon onto sugar-free bread or toast, or for a weight-loss diet onto a large lettuce or cabbage leaf. Fold over or roll up to eat.

Faux Potato Salad

To serve with the sandwich of your choice.

Makes 4 to 6 servings.

1 head cauliflower, broken into florets
½ cup diced scallions
3 chopped celery stalks
3 chopped hard-cooked eggs
salt and pepper to taste

Dressing:
2 teaspoons dry mustard powder
2 tablespoons vinegar
1 cup sugar-free mayonnaise
1 teaspoon celery salt
1 tablespoon snipped fresh dill weed

Steam the cauliflower florets until they are the same texture as boiled potatoes. Assemble the salad ingredients. Allow the cauliflower to cool and add it to the other ingredients. Beat the dressing ingredients until smooth and gently fold into the salad. This salad must be refrigerated for a few hours before serving.

Tuna Salad Variations

Chopped olive
Chopped celery
Chopped radish
Cilantro
Cumin, tomato, and cilantro
Capers

Spoon onto sugar-free bread or toast, or for a weight-loss diet onto a large lettuce or cabbage leaf. Fold over or roll up to eat.

Chicken Salad

Makes 2 to 3 servings.

½ cup mayonnaise
1 teaspoon curry powder
dash of cinnamon
dash of turmeric
dash of cumin
1 teaspoon balsamic vinegar
2 cups cubed chicken
½ cup celery
½ cup peeled and chopped cucumber

Combine all the ingredients. Spoon onto sugar-free bread or toast, or for a weight-loss diet onto a large lettuce or cabbage leaf. Fold over or roll up to eat.

BLT (for weight-loss diet)

Makes 2 "sandwiches."

> 1 head iceberg lettuce
> sugar-free mayonnaise
> 2 ripe tomatoes, chopped
> 6 slices bacon, cooked

Make cups from lettuce leaves. Spread with mayo, and place a small pile of chopped lettuce into each cup. Add some chopped tomatoes, and top with the bacon, broken into pieces. Fold up the lettuce cup to eat.

Spinach, Avocado, and Bacon Salad with Feta

Serves 12.

> 1 16-ounce bag spinach leaves
> 6 scallions, chopped, including green
> ½ cup crumbled feta or chopped goat cheese
> 1 medium avocado, chopped
> 4 slices crisp bacon, crumbled
> 3 tablespoons ground walnuts (grind in a food processor or
>   blender), or whole pine nuts

Combine the salad ingredients in a bowl. In a smaller bowl, whisk together ½ cup extra-virgin olive oil, ½ teaspoon dried mustard, and 2 tablespoons balsamic vinegar. Pour over the salad and toss.

Fried Egg and Goat Cheese Salad

Serves 2.

4 slices thick bacon, chopped
1 tablespoon balsamic vinegar
½ cup olive oil
1 teaspoon Dijon mustard
½ teaspoon dill
½ teaspoon garlic salt
½ teaspoon pepper
1 package (or 6 cups) mixed salad greens (oak leaf lettuce,
    arugula, endive—fancy greens are really nice with this salad)
1 cup crumbled goat cheese or any soft cheese
½ cup pine nuts or chopped walnuts
4 eggs

Cook the bacon until crisp, and remove from the pan. Pour off all but about 1 tablespoon of the bacon grease. In a small bowl, whisk together the vinegar, oil, mustard, dill, garlic salt, and pepper. In a salad bowl, toss together the dressing and the salad greens. Add the crumbled goat cheese and pine nuts, toss, and put onto individual dishes. Reheat the bacon drippings and break the eggs into the pan. Cook until set, and turn over if desired. You can also make this with basted eggs, which seals them: When cooked to desired doneness, instead of turning, pour a spoonful of hot water over the yolk of the egg. Carefully slide the eggs on top of the salad and sprinkle with chopped bacon. A few dried crushed red chilies will look pretty if sprinkled over the eggs with some ground pepper.

Basic Quiche

Makes 1 quiche (6 to 8 servings).

> 6 eggs
> 1 cup heavy cream
> 1 cup grated Swiss cheese

Preheat the oven to 350 degrees. Butter a quiche pan.

Beat the eggs in a bowl with the cream, salt, and pepper. Add the cheese and mix together. Pour into a quiche pan and bake for 40 minutes. Serve hot or cold.

Meat: Add ½ cup ham, sausage, crumbled bacon, or ground beef.

Spinach: Add 1 cup of spinach, cooked and chopped. You can also thaw a package of frozen spinach.

Use Cheddar, Gruyère, or Gouda cheese instead of Swiss.

Stir-Fried Vegetables

> 1 tablespoon peanut oil for each vegetable selected
> 1 garlic clove, chopped, for each vegetable selected
> 2 tablespoons soy sauce
> 2 teaspoons lemon juice
> ½ teaspoon dried mustard
> ½ teaspoon Worcestershire sauce
> ½ teaspoon crushed red pepper flakes
> Vegetables sliced into bite-size pieces, such as zucchini, water chestnuts, leeks, bamboo shoots, radishes, summer squash, asparagus, celery, green beans, mushrooms, and broccoli

Heat 1 tablespoon of peanut oil in a wok on high heat. Add the chopped garlic clove. Stir-fry the first vegetable until softer, but still crunchy. Remove from the pan, add more peanut oil and garlic, and cook the next vegetable. This way each vegetable can be cooked to the proper texture. When all the vegetables have been cooked, return them to the wok and mix together with soy sauce, lemon juice, mustard, and Worcestershire. Sprinkle with crushed red pepper flakes before serving.

DINNER

For many people, dinner doesn't change very much on the HG diet except for removing the starch dish. You'll need to substitute another dish for potatoes, rice, or pasta. Grilled, broiled, or baked meat, fish, or poultry are fine, as long as the seasonings you use don't contain sugar. The vast majority of vegetable dishes don't have to be changed for this diet; just make sure you don't eat any of the forbidden ones. Crock-Pots or slow cookers are wonderful for making easy dinners that will be ready when you get home from work.

Zucchini Fettuccine

Serves 4 as an appetizer, 2 as a main course.

1 cup heavy cream
6 good-size zucchini
1 tablespoon Parmesan or Romano cheese

Put the cream in a saucepan and simmer until reduced by half, about 30 minutes. Cut the zucchini into thin strips using a vegetable peeler. Bring a larger pot full of water to a boil. Drop the zucchini into the boiling water and cook for about 2 minutes. Drain, and toss with a little lemon juice. When the cream has been reduced, add the Parmesan cheese to the cream. Pour the mixture over the zucchini and toss.

You can also top with 1 can diced tomatoes, 1 teaspoon oregano, or chopped Italian sausage. Top with grated Parmesan cheese.

Fish with a Nut Crust (Sea Bass, Sole, Cod)

For this you need to pick a mild fish that comes in a fillet, not a steak. You could also use John Dory or orange roughy, for example.

Serves 4.

½ cup mayonnaise (sugar-free)
½ cup finely chopped almonds or walnuts
1 pound fish fillets

Preheat the oven to 400 degrees. Mix the mayonnaise and nuts and use them to coat the fish. Place the fillets in a single layer on a baking dish or cookie sheet that has been coated with olive oil. Bake for 15 minutes on each side, until golden brown. We put a pat of butter on the final side for the last few minutes of baking. Serve with a lemon wedge.

Spaghetti Squash

Serves 4 as an appetizer, 2 as a main course.

1 spaghetti squash
3 tablespoons butter
½ cup grated Parmesan cheese

Cut the squash in half and put it in a microwave-safe baking dish, cut-side down, with a tablespoon of water. Microwave until tender, about 10 minutes. Take the squash and pull out the strands. Toss the squash with the butter, Parmesan, salt, and pepper. You can also serve with sugar-free marinara sauce or with meat sauce. Top each serving with additional Parmesan cheese.

Roasted Tomatoes

Roasted tomatoes make a good accompaniment for a steak or chicken breast. You can make them in advance and keep in a jar in the refrigerator. These have a very sweet flavor.

Serves 4 as an appetizer or side dish.

> 4 cups cherry tomatoes, cut in half
> 4 garlic cloves, finely chopped

Preheat the oven to 200 degrees. Place the tomatoes and garlic in a baking dish and drizzle with olive oil. You can also make this dish without the garlic for a sweeter flavor, and you can top with chopped basil if you like. Bake in the oven for 2 hours, and serve hot or cold.

Caprese

If you've traveled in Italy, you never forget this dish. It's a wonderful way to start a dinner in summertime, or to have for lunch.

> vine-ripened or home-grown tomatoes, very ripe, sliced
> buffalo mozzarella, sliced
> chopped fresh basil
> olive oil

Lay the tomato slices flat on a plate. On top of each tomato slice, add a slice of mozzarella. Put fresh basil on top, and drizzle with olive oil.

Paola's Steak with Sweet Red Peppers

Simple and wonderful, like the best of Tuscan cooking. You can also use Italian sausage.

> ½ cup olive oil
> 1 pound large red bell peppers, seeded, sliced into ½-inch-thick strips
> garlic salt to taste
> 4 steaks, grilled, broiled, or pan-fried

Heat the oil in a skillet. When it's hot, add the sliced red peppers and garlic salt, cooking until the peppers are soft. Top the steaks with spoonfuls of the peppers.

For steaks, you can also make a topping of sliced elephant garlic or mushrooms sautéed in a little olive oil or butter. To the latter, add ½ cup marsala or white wine.

Fried Chicken

Serves 4.

> ⅓ cup cream
> 2 eggs
> 1½ cups crumbled pork rinds (we do this in the blender)
> 1 pound chicken pieces
> peanut oil, for frying

Mix the cream and eggs in a small bowl. Put the crushed pork rinds on a plate. Dip the chicken pieces in the egg mixture first, then coat with pork rinds. Heat the oil in a heavy skillet and fry the chicken. After the chicken is fried, salt and pepper to taste.

Eggplant Pizza

Serves 2.

1 pound eggplant, cut into $\frac{1}{3}$-inch-thick slices
10 slices pepperoni, or 1 cup cooked ground beef or sausage
1 8-ounce can sugar-free tomato sauce
2 cups grated mozzarella
2 tablespoons grated Parmesan cheese
1 teaspoon oregano, basil, or garlic, chopped fine

Preheat the oven to 425 degrees. Brush the eggplant slices with olive oil on both sides and place on a baking sheet. Bake for 10 minutes and turn; bake 10 minutes more.

Remove from oven. Top each slice with a dollop of tomato sauce, then pepperoni or sausage, then seasonings, mozzarella, and grated Parmesan cheese. Return to oven until sauce is hot and cheese is melted.

Poached Salmon

Serves 4.

$\frac{1}{2}$ cup lemon juice
$\frac{1}{2}$ cup white wine
1 pound salmon steak
$\frac{1}{2}$ cup snipped fresh dill

Preheat the oven to 375 degrees. Place the liquid in a baking dish and lay the salmon in it. Sprinkle the dill on top of the salmon, adding salt and pepper. Cover the dish with a lid or with aluminum foil and bake for 20 minutes.

Serve on a bed of lightly cooked spinach.

Chicken Piccata

Serves 4.

    4 boneless chicken breasts
    6 tablespoons butter
    soy flour
    ½ cup white wine
    ½ cup lemon juice
    1 tablespoon capers

Butterfly the chicken breasts by cutting them in half the long way, to make them thin and wide. Lightly pound them. Heat 2 tablespoons of butter in a skillet. Dust the chicken breasts in soy flour or low-carb baking mix. Add to the skillet and brown both sides. Remove the chicken and set aside. Add the wine, lemon juice, and capers to the skillet and cook over medium heat until the sauce is reduced. Add 4 tablespoons of butter as it cooks. Return the chicken to pan and re-heat it with the sauce. Pour the sauce over the chicken and serve.

Steak au Poivre

Serves 2

    2 tablespoons peppercorns
    2 8-ounce ribeye steaks

2 tablespoons olive oil
1 cup cream
2 tablespoons cognac (or any brandy)

Crush the peppercorns in a blender or with a rolling pin. Press the steaks on top of the peppercorns until they are well coated. Pan-fry the steaks in a heavy skillet with 1 tablespoon of olive oil for each (5 minutes a side will give you medium rare). Remove the steaks from skillet. Add the cream and cognac to the skillet and heat to a boil, stirring and scraping the bottom of the pan as you go. Lower the heat and cook for about 3 minutes, until the sauce is thick. Pour over the steaks and serve.

Angela's Chicken with Creamy Plum Sauce

This recipe comes from Angela Taylor of Oklahoma. It's not for a weight-loss diet.

Serves 2.

2 tablespoons butter
4 boneless chicken breasts, halved
1 cup cream
1 tablespoon Dijon mustard
1 teaspoon crumbled, dried tarragon
2 small plums, halved, pitted, and thinly sliced
3 tablespoons coarsely ground almonds

Heat the butter in a large deep skillet over medium-high heat until the foam subsides. Add the chicken and cook until brown—about 3 minutes on each side. Add the cream to the skillet. Bring to a gentle boil, lower the heat, and simmer for 6 minutes, turning the chicken several times. Stir the cream as well so it doesn't burn. Stir in the mustard, tarragon, salt, pepper, and plums, making sure to coat the chicken. Cook over medium heat for 3 minutes. Remove from the heat and stir in the almonds. Serve immediately.

Vegetable Puree with Garlic

Serves 2 to 4 as a side dish.

    3 heads broccoli or cauliflower, broken into florets (you can
        also use fennel, red bell peppers, or leeks)
    4 garlic cloves
    ½ cup heavy cream

Steam the vegetables until soft in the microwave or in a pot. Combine with the garlic, cream, salt, and pepper in a food processor. Puree for about 2 minutes, until smooth.

Baked Spinach

Serves 4 as a side dish.

    1 cup whole-milk ricotta or cottage cheese
    ½ teaspoon white Worcestershire sauce
    2 eggs
    1 (10-ounce) package chopped frozen spinach
    2 teaspoons caraway seeds
    3 tablespoons chopped walnuts
    ½ cup grated Cheddar cheese (sharp is best)

Preheat the oven to 350 degrees. Combine the ricotta with a dash of salt and pepper and the Worcestershire sauce in a blender. Blend until smooth, adding the eggs as you go. Combine this mixture with the spinach, seeds, and nuts in a baking pan and sprinkle the Cheddar over the top. Bake for 25 minutes.

Cauliflower Soufflés

You could also substitute zucchini or (on a liberal diet) carrots for the cauliflower in this recipe.

Makes 10 small soufflés.

> 2 cups cauliflower
> ½ cup chopped scallions, shallots, or white onion (on a liberal diet)
> 2 eggs
> 1 teaspoon baking powder
> 1 tablespoon soy flour
> 1 teaspoon salt or garlic salt

Preheat the oven to 325 degrees. Grease 10 muffin cups with oil or nonstick spray.

Combine all the ingredients in a blender or food processor and blend well. The mixture should be smooth. Pour into muffin tins; do not overfill. Bake for 20 minutes, until light brown.

These are nice served with sour cream and curry powder (whisked together to taste) or Dijon mustard.

Green Beans Amandine

Serves 2 as a side dish.

> ½ cup slivered blanched almonds
> ½ cup butter
> ½ teaspoon salt
> 1 teaspoon lemon juice
> 2 cups cooked green beans (thawed frozen, canned at room temperature, or fresh beans that have been lightly steamed in the microwave for 1 minute).

Cook the almonds in the butter over medium heat until golden. Add the salt and lemon juice. Add the green beans to the pan and toss gently.

Lou's Superbowl Chili

For weight loss, you can omit the onion garnish, and use chopped shallot, scallions, or leeks instead.

Serves 4.

1 pound ground chuck
2 small onions, chopped fine
4 garlic cloves, chopped fine
½ cup sugar-free tomato sauce
½ cup tomato paste (no sugar added)
1 cup water
1 tablespoon red wine vinegar
½ teaspoon white vinegar
½ teaspoon ground allspice
1 bay leaf
½ teaspoon cayenne pepper
1 tablespoon chili powder
1 teaspoon ground black pepper
½ teaspoon cardamom
½ teaspoon ground cloves
½ teaspoon cumin
½ teaspoon turmeric
½ teaspoon mace
½ teaspoon marjoram
1 teaspoon onion powder
1 tablespoon paprika
1 teaspoon salt
1 ounce unsweetened baking chocolate

Heat a large, heavy skillet until hot, and then add and brown the meat. When the meat is nearly cooked, add the onions and garlic. Then add the tomato sauce and paste, the water, and the vinegars. Heat until the mixture begins to boil and then add the spices, including the chocolate. Cover the chili and simmer over very low heat for about 1 hour, stirring occasionally to make sure it doesn't stick to the bottom of the pan. If the mixture gets too thick while cooking, add some beef bouillon as needed. Top with grated cheese, chopped onion, and a dollop of sour cream if desired.

Cheesy Mixed Vegetables

Serves 2 as a main course, 4 as a side dish.

    4 cups chopped vegetables: eggplant, cabbage, summer
       squash, mushrooms, celery, brussels sprouts, cauliflower,
       leeks, broccoli, green beans, asparagus spears, peppers
       (red, green, or yellow), onions (liberal diet), tomatoes
       (seeded), okra, etc.
    2 cups grated cheese: Gruyère, Cheddar, Jack, Swiss, Muenster

Steam the vegetables on the stovetop or in a microwave. You should do this in batches, mixing the harder vegetables together, and the softer ones together. Keep the vegetables crisp but soft enough to chew. Put the vegetables in a bowl and mix, then cover with the cheese. If the warm vegetables don't melt the cheese, then put them under the broiler for a minute.

Crock-Pot Brisket

Serves 4.

> 3–4 pound brisket
> 1 teaspoon garlic salt
> 1 teaspoon celery salt
> 1 teaspoon dry mustard
> ½ teaspoon dried rosemary
> ½ cup Liquid Smoke

Heat the oven to broil. When the oven is hot, place the roast in the center on a cookie sheet, and cook for 10 minutes. Some fat will cook off, and the brisket will brown. Remove from the oven and place on a large piece of aluminum foil. Sprinkle with the spices and Liquid Smoke. Wrap the brisket well and put it into a Crock-Pot. Cook on low for 10 hours (or high for 6). Serve sliced thinly, with pot juice poured over it.

Leek and Meatball Casserole

This casserole can be made ahead of time and refrigerated. It takes about 10 minutes to heat in a broiler to serve.

Serves 4.

> ½ pound ground beef
> ½ teaspoon paprika
> 3 garlic cloves, sliced finely
> 3 leeks, washed and cut into ½-inch-thick slices
> 2 cups finely chopped cauliflower
> ½ cup celery cut into ½-inch slices
> 1 tablespoon olive oil
> 1 tablespoon butter

1 cup grated sharp Cheddar cheese
½ cup pork rinds, crushed
2 tablespoons Parmesan cheese

Preheat the broiler.

Form the ground beef into bite-size meatballs and brown in a frying pan. After the meatballs are brown, sprinkle with paprika and half of the garlic and cook until cooked through. Remove from the pan and set aside. Carefully trim off the outer leaves of the leeks and cut off the nontender green parts. You can leave on as much of the stem as looks tender and fresh. Chop the cauliflower to the size of uncooked rice. Cut the celery into ½-inch slices. In the frying pan, heat the olive oil and add the butter. Add the sliced leeks and the rest of the garlic and cook for about 4 minutes, until they are starting to soften up. Then add the chopped celery and cauliflower and cook until the leeks are tender. (The celery and cauliflower will be crunchy.) In an oven-proof pan, spoon together the vegetable mixture and the meatballs. Season with pepper to taste. Cover the mixture with a layer of grated Cheddar cheese and sprinkle with crushed pork rinds. Place under the broiler until the cheese is melted and starting to brown. When serving, sprinkle with Parmesan cheese and a sugar-free salsa or hot sauce, if desired. For dinner, add a green salad with a mild dressing—the casserole is rich.

Faux Tatoes

There are two ways to make mashed potatoes on the low-carbohydrate diet, and both are fine for weight loss as well. The first is to use cauliflower and the second is to use celery root (celeriac).

Cauliflower Faux Tatoes

Serves 2.

Break a head of cauliflower apart into florets, and steam or microwave until they are very soft. Put into a food processor and puree, adding cream and butter to taste. You can also use a mixture of sour cream and heavy cream. Salt and pepper to taste. Some recipes also use cream cheese and butter. Blue cheese makes a nice addition, too.

Celery Root (Celeriac) Faux Tatoes

Celery root is easily found in most markets, near the fennel, leeks, and daikon. Usually about the size of a baseball, it's white with brown knots and hairy roots. To prepare: Wash carefully, use a knife to trim away the roots, and then peel. Chop into chunks to steam for faux tatoes, or cut up like french fries and cook in hot oil to make faux fries. Some cooks soak it in water before cooking with it, but this is not necessary.

Each root serves 2.

Steam the celery root in the microwave or on top of the stove until soft. Transfer to a blender and puree, adding cream, butter, salt, and pepper to taste. Sour cream and cream cheese (or other cheese) can be added to taste as well.

Faux Tato Croquettes

Makes 2 to 4 servings.

   1 recipe faux tatoes
   2 eggs, beaten

1 large package pork rinds, crushed in a blender
paprika, for garnish

Refrigerate the faux tatoes until cold and firm. Form the mixture into 1½-inch balls, and dip each ball into the beaten eggs. Roll in the crushed pork rinds. Fry a few croquettes at a time in cooking oil. Remove from the heat when brown, and set on paper towels to drain. When serving, sprinkle with paprika. You can make these in batches and freeze them. Reheat in the oven at 350 degrees for 30 minutes or until hot through.

Chicken-Fried Steak

Serves 4.

2 eggs
1 cup crushed pork rinds (you can put them in the blender)
1 tablespoon soy protein powder
4 cube steaks
3 tablespoons oil, for frying
2 cups cauliflower, steamed until very soft
⅓ cup heavy cream
½ cup beef bouillon
1 teaspoon salt
1 teaspoon pepper

Beat the eggs until frothy. Put the crushed pork rinds and soy powder on a plate, and mix together well. Soak the steaks in the eggs until covered, and then press well into the pork rind mixture, coating the meat on both sides. When all the steaks are coated, heat the oil in a skillet until hot. Cook the steaks until they are brown and crispy on both sides. While the steaks are cooking, put the cauliflower and cream into the blender and whip until smooth. When the steaks are done, add the bouillon to the pan you cooked them in, scraping the pan drippings into it. Pour this mixture back into a heatproof measuring cup. Turn the blender back on and slowly add the salt and pepper, then the bouillon mixture. You may not need to use it all. When the contents of the blender are the consistency of cream gravy, stop adding the liquid. If the mixture isn't hot, you can heat it in the skillet or microwave. Pour over the steaks and serve.

Shepherd's Pie

Serves 4.

    1 pound ground beef
    ½ teaspoon oregano
    1 bay leaf
    1 cup chopped mushrooms
    2 garlic cloves, chopped
    ½ cup sour cream
    3 cups faux tatoes
    ½ cup shredded cheese (Jack, Swiss, or Cheddar)

Preheat the oven to 350 degrees. Brown the beef with the spices in a skillet and drain. Remove the bay leaf. Microwave or sauté the mushrooms with the garlic until soft, and add to the ground meat. Add the sour cream to this and mix well. Prepare the faux tatoes (you can use leftovers)—you need about 3 cups. Spread on the bottom of a baking dish. Spoon the meat mixture over this layer. Top with grated cheese and bake for 30 minutes.

Tarragon Chicken Breasts

Serves 4.

    3 tablespoons butter
    6 boneless chicken breasts (can be skinless if desired)

½ cup chopped leeks (the white part) or scallions
½ cup white wine, sherry, or vermouth
3 tablespoons Dijon mustard
½ cup heavy cream
3 tablespoons chopped fresh tarragon
1 tablespoon chopped fresh parsley

Melt the butter in a skillet over medium heat. When bubbly, add the chicken breasts, along with salt and pepper. Cook until the chicken is completely done, about 5 minutes a side. Remove the chicken from the pan, add the leeks, and cook until soft. Add the wine and mustard and simmer while scraping the pan. Add the cream, tarragon, and parsley, and cook until the sauce is thick, stirring continually. Pour the sauce over the chicken and serve.

SNACKS

On the liberal diet, the snacks we've listed include things like protein bars, shakes, and other prepackaged foods. Beware of these foods on the weight-loss diet, however, since they contain hidden carbohydrates. They are also expensive and should be used in moderation due to their sugar alcohols, which can cause gas and other intestinal symptoms.

Cucumber Finger Sandwiches

Serves 4.

4 English cucumbers (the long hothouse variety)
1 cup crab, lobster, chicken, or egg salad with 1 teaspoon of
    snipped dill added
paprika, for garnish

Peel the cucumbers and slice them in half lengthwise. Scoop out the seeds and place spoonfuls of the salad into the center. Slice the cucumbers in half or thirds, and sprinkle with paprika.

You can also fill celery stalks with the same salad mixture.

Roast Beef or Ham Roll-Ups

Serves 2.

6 slices roast beef, ham, or turkey meat (3 per roll-up)
½ cup cream cheese
1 teaspoon grated horseradish (or pesto, chopped red peppers, celery, olive paste, chopped nuts, mustard, or ½ teaspoon curry powder)

Place a slice of roast beef on a plate. Mix together well the cream cheese and horseradish. Spread thickly on the roast beef, and roll up.

Vegetable Slices

Daikon—cut into ½-inch slices and drip lime juice on them. Sprinkle with salt.
Jicama—cut into slices ½ inch thick and add a drop of lemon or lime juice. Sprinkle with chili pepper or Pico de Gallo.
Watermelon radish—slice into rounds and use as a cracker with cream cheese.

Traditional Deviled Eggs

Cut cold hard-boiled eggs in half.

Remove the yolks and mash them with 2 teaspoons of sugar-free mayonnaise, salt, and pepper to taste for each egg. Fill the hole in the egg whites with the mixture, and garnish with paprika. Add dry mustard, cumin, curry powder, smoked salmon, or capers to the egg yolks for variety.

Crunchy Cheese Crackers

This works with any drier cheese that you can grate coarsely. You can use Parmesan, Romano, sharp Cheddar, Gouda, Edam, and more.

Grate the cheese. Heat the broiler. Spray a baking sheet with a nonstick coating such as Pam or a thin film of cooking oil (you don't need much). Place tablespoon-size heaps of cheese on the baking sheet about an inch apart. Put under the broiler 3 inches from the heat. When the cheese is bubbly, remove the baking sheet and let it cool for a few minutes. Remove the crackers with a spatula and dry on paper towels to absorb the grease.

Quick Pepperoni Chips

Place slices of pepperoni on a paper towel. Cover with a second paper towel and microwave until crisp; the time will vary depending on how many chips you are making and how powerful your microwave is. The chips come out crispy, with the fat cooked off. You can eat these with cheese, or crumble them into salads, soups, or what have you.

Celery Snacks

Fill celery stalks with a mixture of equal parts blue cheese and butter, mashed together. Sprinkle with chopped walnuts.

Quick Green Bean Salad

Keep a can of green beans in the refrigerator just for this salad. Open the can and drain the beans. Toss with red wine vinegar to taste, adding a dash of garlic salt and olive oil if desired.

Hot Dips

Serves 4.

- 2 cups chopped chicken, salmon, or crabmeat
- ½ cup sugar-free mayonnaise
- ½ cup grated Swiss, Cheddar, or Jack cheese
- ½ cup grated Parmesan cheese
- ½ teaspoon salt
- ½ teaspoon pepper
- dash of cayenne pepper
- dash of garlic salt
- 2 chopped scallions, green part and all
- ½ teaspoon whichever spice you like best (we like dill with salmon, cumin or tarragon with chicken, thyme or horseradish with crab)

Preheat the oven to 350 degrees. Mix together all the ingredients and spread in a buttered baking dish. Bake for 10 minutes, until the top is brown, and cut into pieces.

Bacon-Wrapped Shrimp

There are several variations on this recipe. You can also put a piece of jalapeño pepper on the shrimp before they're wrapped with the bacon; these are called Cowboy Kisses. You can obviously make as many of these as you like.

Makes 2 to 4 servings.

10 cooked large shrimp (if frozen, you can thaw in the microwave)
1 tablespoon chopped basil (or herb of your choice)
2 tablespoons balsamic vinegar
10 slices bacon (partially cook this in the microwave wrapped in a paper towel if you like your bacon well done)
crumbled blue or Gorgonzola cheese, or sharp white Cheddar

Preheat the oven to broil.

Arrange the shrimp in a single layer on a cookie sheet. Sprinkle them with the chopped herbs and top each with a dash of balsamic vinegar. You can also add a dash of cayenne pepper, crushed red chili peppers, or a slice of jalapeño pepper. Wrap each shrimp with a slice of bacon and hold it in place with a toothpick. Broil until the bacon is cooked. Transfer to a plate and sprinkle with crumbled cheese.

Root Beer Float

⅓ cup heavy cream
1 can diet root beer

Whip the heavy cream until thick. Pour into a tall glass, and add the root beer.

Baked Apples

These also make a nice dessert or even a breakfast dish.

Serves 4.

> 4 large tart apples
> ½ cup Splenda (or the equivalent amount of liquid sweetener)
> 1 tablespoon cinnamon
> ½ cup chopped pecans, walnuts, or almonds
> about 1 teaspoon grated lemon rind
> 4 teaspoons butter (more if desired)
> 2 tablespoons Splenda or liquid sweetener

Preheat the oven to 375 degrees. Wash and core the apples. Do not cut through to bottom; leave ½ inch of apple below the core. Combine the ½ cup of sweetener, nuts, and cinnamon. Add ⅛ teaspoon grated lemon rind. Fill the apple centers with a spoonful of this mixture, and cover with a pat of butter. Put the apples into a baking dish that has ½ cup of boiling water in it, with 2 tablespoons of sugar substitute added to it. (You can also use Da Vinci sugar-free cinnamon or caramel syrup.) Bake for 40 to 60 minutes, until the apples are tender. Remove the apples from the dish and put into individual serving dishes. Baste with the juice from the pan. Serve hot or cold, garnished with a dab of whipped cream.

Protein Shake I

Makes 1 16-ounce shake.

1½ cups prepared Crystal Light
½ cup heavy cream
1 tablespoon sour cream
1 tablespoon cream cheese
1 cup ice cubes

Put the ingredients in a blender and mix well.

Protein Shake II

Makes 1 16-ounce shake.

1 can sugar-free orange, grape, or chocolate soda
2 scoops vanilla-flavor protein powder or 2 scoops protein
powder and 1 teaspoon vanilla extract
½ cup heavy cream
1 cup ice cubes

Put the ingredients in a blender and mix well.

DESSERTS

Given the wide choice of nonsugar sweeteners on the market, there's a lot you can make for dessert. Nuts, cream, cream cheese, and sugar-free Jell-O can be used in many combinations. If you have an ice cream maker, you can certainly make delicious ice cream. For weight loss, be sure to watch quantities. It's best to treat these desserts as treats. Many companies also have low-carbohydrate baking mixes available.

Peaches Flambé

You can also use pears in this recipe. It's not for a weight-loss diet.

Ripe peaches, cut in half
2 teaspoons butter per peach
1 teaspoon Splenda per peach
½ cup brandy per peach
1 tablespoon whipped cream per peach
1 teaspoon chopped pecans or walnuts per peach

Preheat the broiler. Place the peaches in a shallow baking pan. Microwave for 30 seconds, or until soft. Remove from the microwave, place a dollop of butter on each half, and top with sugar substitute. Place under the broiler until lightly brown. Place the peaches in a heatproof serving dish, and pour brandy over them. Light the brandy and allow the alcohol to burn off. Top with whipped cream and 1 teaspoon crushed nuts.

Piecrust

½ cup low-carb baking mix (Atkins)
2 tablespoons Splenda
½ cup heavy cream
1 egg
1 teaspoon vanilla extract

Preheat the oven to 350 degrees. Whisk together the dry ingredients in a small mixing bowl. Add the cream, eggs, and vanilla extract. Beat until smooth. Let the mixture set for 10 minutes.

Spread mixture in a pie pan and bake until set and browned.

Creamy Pie Filling

Fills 1 9-inch pie crust.

8 ounces softened cream cheese
5 teaspoons Splenda
1 teaspoon butterscotch or almond extract
1 cup heavy cream
1 teaspoon vanilla extract

In a small bowl, cream the cream cheese, 4 teaspoons of the Splenda, and the butterscotch or almond extract. Set aside. In a larger bowl, mix together the heavy cream, vanilla, and remaining 1 teaspoon of Splenda. Beat until very stiff. Then fold in the cream cheese mixture and mix well, but gently. Pour into a cooled piecrust. Chill before serving.

Pudding Filling (or Just Pudding)

Fills 1 9-inch piecrust or 4 pudding cups.

5 eggs
3 egg yolks, beaten
½ cup Splenda
1 tablespoon vanilla extract
2 cups heavy cream
nutmeg or cinnamon

Preheat the oven to 325 degrees. Whisk together the eggs and egg yolks. When well beaten, add the Splenda and cream. Pour into a pie shell or ovenproof dish and bake for 30 minutes. When cool, sprinkle with cinnamon or nutmeg.

Gwen's Baked Custard

This recipe is also good for breakfast and snacks.

Makes 6 servings.

>   2 cups cream
>   2 eggs
>   2 tablespoons Splenda
>   ½ teaspoon imitation vanilla (with no alcohol)
>   ⅛ teaspoon salt
>   ground nutmeg (optional)

Preheat the oven to 350 degrees. Using an electric mixer, beat together all ingredients until very well blended. Fill six 5-ounce custard
cups. Sprinkle each with a light dusting of ground nutmeg. Place the
cups in a 9 x 13 x 2 cake pan in the middle of the preheated oven.
Pour boiling water into the cake pan, 1 inch deep. Bake for 40 minutes or until a knife inserted off center comes out clean. Serve warm
or chilled. To unmold the chilled custard, first loosen the edge with a
knife, then slip the point of the knife down the side to let air in. Invert
onto small dessert dish and garnish with a dollop of whipped cream
and a sliced strawberry, if desired.

Delicious and Anonymous Cheesecake

*This is the easiest and best cheesecake recipe we've seen. It requires
no springform pan or hot-water bath. A patient gave it to us one day
in the office. Unfortunately, she did not write her name on the paper,
and we couldn't remember who gave it to us. We called every patient
we thought might be responsible, but couldn't find the author.
Thanks, whoever you are!*

Cheesecake:
12 ounces cream cheese (1½ cups)
½ cup Splenda
1 teaspoon vanilla extract
2 beaten egg yolks
2 stiffly beaten egg whites

Topping:
2 cups sour cream
4 tablespoons Splenda

Preheat the oven to 350 degrees. Mix together the cream cheese, Splenda, vanilla, and egg yolks. When the mixture is a creamy texture, fold in the egg whites. Pour into an unbaked nut crust (see the next recipe). Bake for 30 minutes. Remove from the oven and let cool. The cheesecake will be puffy, but as it cools it will shrink down. Make the topping by mixing together the sour cream and Splenda until creamy. When the cheesecake is cool, pour this mixture over the top. Turn the oven up to 375 degrees, and bake for 5 more minutes. Cool in the refrigerator until ready to eat.

Basic Nut Crust

On the strict side of the diet, only 1 slice of this crust is acceptable, and it uses up your nut allowance for the day. You can decrease the amount of nuts in the recipe by using half nuts and half no-carbohydrate baking mix such at Atkins or Carbolyte.

1½ cups pecans or walnuts, chopped very fine in a food
    processor or blender
2 tablespoons melted butter
2 tablespoons Splenda
1 egg white, beaten until frothy

Mix together the nuts, butter, and Splenda. Then fold in the egg white and mix until all the nuts are moistened. Pat into an 8-inch pie pan and set aside.

Jeri Lynn's Tonga Lime Soufflé

5 eggs, separated
1 cup Splenda
2 teaspoons grated lime rind
½ cup lime juice
1 tablespoon gelatin
⅓ cup warm water
½ cup cream, lightly whipped

Beat the egg yolks, Splenda, and lime rind for 3 minutes, until the mixture is thick and pale. Heat the lime juice and very slowly add the egg yolk mixture while beating. Combine the gelatin in a small bowl with warm water to soften. Stir until the gelatin is dissolved. Add the gelatin gradually to the lime mixture, and beat until combined. Transfer to a larger bowl and cover with plastic wrap. Refrigerate for 15 minutes until thickened but not set. Use a spatula to fold in the whipped cream. Whip the egg whites to soft peaks and combine with the lime mixture. Spoon gently into individual ramekins and chill.

Dessert Crepes with Strawberry Filling

You can use a mixture of berries, within the daily limit—very delicious. This dish, made with strawberries, is acceptable for a weight-loss diet.

Makes 4 large crepes.

Crepes:
1 egg, well beaten
3 tablespoons whole-milk ricotta
1 teaspoon vanilla extract
heavy dash of cinnamon
heavy dash of nutmeg
2 tablespoons Splenda
1 teaspoon butter or margarine

Filling:
1 cup sour cream

Blend together the crepe ingredients. The batter will be thin. Heat the butter or margarine in a crepe or nonstick pan. Pour in enough mixture to cover the bottom of the pan in a thin layer. Let cook until set—the crepe should slide around when you move the pan. Flip one time and brown the second side. This is tricky. (You can slide the crepe out of the pan onto a paper plate, and then slide it back in by turning the plate.) Top with sour cream and slices of strawberry. Roll up and garnish with a dollop of sour cream and a slice of berry.

Crème Fraiche and Strawberries

You can also buy crème fraiche in markets, but it is inexplicably expensive. You have to plan this at least 24 hours in advance, but it will keep for about a week. It makes a good snack or breakfast on a warm day.

Makes 2 to 4 servings.

1 cup sour cream
1 cup heavy cream
dash of vanilla extract

Whisk together the ingredients until well blended and a little thick. Set out at room temperature for 24 hours. Then chill before serving. Serve with your daily portion of strawberries.

Crème Fraiche Ice Cream

Cream 8 egg yolks with 1 cup of Splenda and 1½ teaspoons of vanilla extract. Add this to 3 cups of crème fraiche and pour into a medium saucepan. Heat over a medium flame until the mixture starts to thicken. Remove from the heat and chill, then use an ice cream maker as directed.

Coconut Macaroons

Makes a dozen cookies.

   2 egg whites
   ½ teaspoon vanilla
   ½ cup Splenda
   ½ cup fine ground nuts (use a blender or food processor)
   1 cup shredded coconut (unsweetened)

Preheat the oven to 350 degrees. Beat the egg whites and vanilla until they're stiff and peaks form. Slowly add the Splenda. Gently fold in the nuts and coconut. Drop 1 teaspoon at a time onto a nonstick cookie sheet, or use a baking sheet covered with parchment paper. Bake until light brown, about 15 minutes.

Basic Vanilla Ice Cream

Many ice creams can be made or adapted to our diet. We're converts: Usually we don't advise buying expensive equipment, but an ice cream maker is well worth it on this diet. You can also make slushes with sugar-free drinks such as Crystal Light.

Serves 4.

> 2½ cups heavy cream
> ½ cup water
> 1 tablespoon vanilla extract
> 4 teaspoons Splenda
> 8 egg yolks

In a saucepan, heat ½ cup of the heavy cream with the vanilla and egg yolks. Heat well, but do not bring to a boil. Slowly add the remaining cream, water, and Splenda and continue to heat. When the mixture is steaming but not boiling, remove from the heat and pour into a bowl. Chill well for at least 2 hours. This mixture is ready for your ice cream maker when it is chilled.

Popsicles

Makes 8 to 10 Popsicles.

> 1 small plastic tub Crystal Light drink mix
> 1 package sugar-free Jell-O
> 2 cups boiling water
> 2 cups cold water

Combine the Crystal Light and Jell-O. Add the boiling water and stir until both have completely dissolved. Add the cold water. Pour into Popsicle makers or ice cube trays and freeze.

Peanut Butter Cheesecake

1½ cups heavy cream
½ cup Splenda
⅓ cup unsweetened peanut butter
½ cup cream cheese

Whip the heavy cream with the Splenda until stiff. Fold in the peanut butter gently, and then the cream cheese. Spoon into a nut crust and chill before serving.

Lana Trotter's Pumpkin Custard

Makes 6 servings.

4 eggs, slightly beaten
1 large can Libby's solid-pack pumpkin
1½ cups Splenda
1 teaspoon salt
½ teaspoon ginger
½ teaspoon ground cloves
1 teaspoon nutmeg
1 teaspoon cinnamon
1 can undiluted Carnation evaporated milk
1½ cups whipping cream

Preheat the oven to 325 degrees. Combine the ingredients in the order listed, and beat together until well mixed. Pour into a glass 9 x 13 baking dish. Bake for 1 hour, until a knife inserted near the center comes out clean. Serve with garnish of whipped cream, or whipped cream and wet walnut sauce. You can also add dark rum and sugar substitute to taste to whipping cream, for a holiday flavor.

Sweet Italian Dessert Cake

Cake:
2 eggs, separated
1 teaspoon vanilla extract
1 teaspoon rum extract
2 cups whole-milk ricotta cheese
1 cup Splenda or other granulated sweetener
½ cup whipping cream
2 tablespoons lemon juice

Glaze:
1 tablespoon Splenda
½ cup sour cream
½ teaspoon rum

Preheat the oven to 350 degrees. Grease a 10-inch glass baking pan. Beat the egg whites and extracts until soft peaks form. Beat together the ricotta, Splenda, cream, and lemon juice until foamy. Gently fold in the egg whites. Pour into the baking dish and bake for 1½ hours. Beat together glaze ingredients and set aside. Remove the cake from the oven and spread the glaze over the top. Return to the oven for 5 minutes, or until the glaze sets. Serve hot or cold, with or without sliced fruit.

FESTIVE AND HOLIDAY TIPS

There are certainly many wonderful holiday dishes that can be made on our diet, and there are also some cookbooks listed in the resource section to help with special occasions. Below are some ideas to get you thinking in a positive way about what you can look forward to.

St. Patrick's Day: Of course not everyone celebrates this one, but corned beef and cabbage are traditional, and you can substitute celery root for potatoes.

Easter/Passover: The spring holidays with their fresh new vegetables make it easy. Lamb can be cooked as usual, but for ham try sugar-free maple syrup instead of honey as a coating. Kugel can be made with cauliflower instead of potato; scalloped potatoes should be replaced with scalloped faux tatoes!

Memorial Day: If you barbecue, you've got no problems. Coleslaw can be made with Splenda (or any sugar substitute), and faux tato salad is another acceptable side. You can even make french fries from celery root if you prefer. Grilled vegetables can be a colorful addition to your meal.

The *Fourth of July* is another holiday on which barbecues and picnics are traditional. Once again, this means grilled meats and vegetables, all of which are acceptable on the diet. Salad ingredients are plentiful this time of year; just load them up with the permissible vegetables and use a sugar-free dressing.

Labor Day: The end of the summer can be celebrated at the beach, where grilled fish and salads can make a wonderful meal. Seafood kabobs can be strung together to order with sweet red and yellow peppers, tomatoes, and red onions (omit the onions for a weight-loss diet). Garlic olive oil and a squirt of balsamic vinegar will bring out the flavor. It's an American holiday, so we've included an American dessert. If you're on the strict diet, though, have strawberries and crème fraiche instead.

Thanksgiving: You can absolutely do this meal low carbohydrate without problems. Make faux tatoes and roast turkey. Make cranberry sauce from scratch using the recipe on the bag, and substituting Splenda for the sugar. Faux yams are easy, too: Microwave a butternut squash until it's soft, and scoop the flesh out of the rind. Put in a glass baking dish and cover with sugar-free maple syrup and crumbled walnuts. When serving, you can even put a dollop of whipped cream on top. You can make turkey stuffing from vegetables, but you can also make faux rice stuffing by chopping cauliflower, water chestnuts, and mushrooms. Add sugar-free bread crumbs (or, for the strict diet, pork rinds) as well as sage and other spices.

Christmas/Winter Holidays: The winter holidays with all the goodies piled around are a difficult time to stick to your diet. Make sure you bring your own goodies if you are worried. Little plastic containers can hold a lot and get you through.

FAST FOOD/ON THE ROAD

> I printed out the diet on one sheet of paper and I carry it in my purse and keep one on the refrigerator door. This way I am never confused no matter how bad my fibrofog is, and I always know what I can eat.
>
> *Shelley K., Los Angeles, California*

Fast-food companies *are* catching on to the low-carbohydrate diets, though perhaps slowly. On the West Coast, we have In N Out—a hamburger place that serves protein burgers in which the meat is wrapped with tomato and onions in a lettuce leaf. Chicken places have baked or broiled chicken entrées and now serve green salads as well.

You can always take the bread off burgers, and have a salad without the dressings that may contain sugar. Most places do have lemon for iced tea. Unfortunately, this era of supersize and jumbo meals doesn't apply to the meat portion of your meal. This doesn't mean you can't get by; it just means it may be difficult to get a lot of food for an inexpensive price.

On any diet, when you travel it's always easier if you carry your own snacks and food to round out what might be skimpy meals without the heavy starches. On the weight-loss diet, this will mean cut-up vegetables, hard-boiled eggs, nuts, and cheese. You can buy string cheese in individual servings, as well as chopped vegetables and cold cuts. Since most supermarkets now have delis and food service, a market might be a better stop than a burger place if you're on the road.

If you travel by car, don't forget that it's easy enough to pick up an inexpensive cooler for your backseat. You can fill plastic bags with food in sensible quantities, buy individual containers of sugar-free Jell-O or cream cheese, and carry your own bread and other staples. Traveling is not a good time to wing it, hoping that there will be something to eat, or making mistakes because you're hungry. Remember that although it may take a little extra time, you'll want to feel your best and not ruin your vacation with fatigue, irritable bowel, or a miserable headache!

COOKING ON YOUR OWN

For three weeks the diet was very difficult. I had carbohydrate cravings, irritability, and headaches. That's how I knew I really needed the diet! After that I felt much better: more energy, less pain, and no cravings. Two years later I find it easy to stay on the diet (with the help of an occasional treat made with sucralose) and am rarely tempted to cheat. The improvement I feel is much better than the temporary pleasure I get from eating pasta or pastry.

Nancy B., Cleveland, Ohio

Now it's time to try your hand at cooking some of *your* favorite foods. It's probably easier than you think, and many recipes don't need any changes. Meat, fish, and poultry main dishes, for example, are usually fine as written. Many vegetable recipes are, too. For some, you'll need a little help. Here are some of the ideas we've devised.

Recipe Substitutions

Cornstarch/Flour (thickening): Try unflavored gelatin or gluten, soy flour, a dash of protein powder, or water chestnuts (put in blender). You can also use a beaten egg yolk or cream to thicken a sauce. With soups, stews, or Crock-Pot dishes, you can also pour the liquid and vegetables or some cooked cauliflower into the blender and blend for a minute to make a thicker mixture. NotStarch can be purchased from Web sites; it takes some practice to use.

Rice: As part of a stuffing or casserole, substitute a mixture of finely chopped (the consistency of rice) raw cauliflower and water chestnuts.

Bread crumbs: For small amounts, make these from sugar-free bread (just toast it or dry it in the oven, then put it in the blender). You can mix with pork rinds (put in the blender or food processor). For larger amounts, you'll need more pork rinds, so you don't overdo it with the bread. You can also make a blend of pork rinds and soy flour or gluten—but watch the soy flour on light meats such as veal, because you can taste it. (For the weight-loss diet, you'll have to use pork rinds, period.) For fish and chicken you can also use crushed nuts.

Potatoes: Substitute steamed cauliflower or steamed celery root. Steam until soft and put into the blender with cream and butter (or sour cream). Use to top casseroles or eat as a side dish with meat or other main dishes.

Whole milk: Substitute 1 part heavy cream and 1 part water for a strict diet, with a dash of Splenda to make sweet.

Onion: For the weight-loss diet only, substitute onion powder (2 teaspoons = ½ cup onions in flavor). Or use leeks or scallions in recipes where you need the volume or texture.

Sugar Substitutes

- *Stevia* has almost no carbohydrates but varies in sweetness. It may also have a bitter aftertaste. You can't use it for baking because it changes the proportions of wet-dry ingredients and volumes. Use in shakes, tea, or other liquids for best results.
- *Splenda* (sucralose) measures the same as sugar. It is natural—it's made from sugar. You can cook with it just like sugar, and it has no aftertaste. It also does not have the side effects (like headaches) that the chemical sweeteners (particularly aspartame) may cause in some people. It does contain carbohydrates—if you are on a strict diet, watch the quantity. If you're trying to lose weight, ½ cup (cumulative over a day) is your entire day's allotment of carbohydrate. Be sure to include gum, breath mints, Rolaids, and the like in this total. (One teaspoon equals ½ gram of carbohydrate. Each packet is 1 gram; 1 cup is 24 grams.)
- *Liquid sweeteners* (Sweet'N Low): Saccharin has an aftertaste, familiar to all who have tried sugar substitutes. It's difficult to cook with because the volume is different than sugar's, but it can certainly be used for protein drinks, custards, and hot drinks. Liquid sugar substitutes have no

dextrose (or other sugars) added, so they have *no* carbohydrates. If you are very sensitive to carbohydrates and trying to lose weight, use liquids wherever possible to keep your total carbohydrates down.

- *Cyclamate* may soon be legal in the United States again; it's used in all other parts of the world in diet products, including sodas. It has no aftertaste, and can be used for cooking. (Cyclamate can be purchased from Canada and is useful for weight loss because it has no carbohydrates.) Since it is not commonly used in the United States, it does not appear in the table below, but ½ teaspoon of it is equivalent to 1 teaspoon of sugar, while ½ cup equals 1 cup of sugar.

- *Equal and NutraSweet* (aspartame) packets do not work well for cooking because they lose sweetness in heating, but they do fine in dressings, shakes, and so on. They each have almost 1 gram of carb per packet, so same warnings apply as for Splenda if you're on a weight-loss diet. Equal Spoonful comes in bulk.

- *AlternaSweet or Sweet One* (acesulfame potassium) can be used for cooking, and like sucralose carries no health warnings.

- *DiabetiSweet* (acesulfame and isomalt) is a synergistic blend of nonsugar sweeteners that can be used for cooking. These "sweet" products have about 4½ grams of carbohydrate *per teaspoon*.

- *Somersweet* is a new sweetener marketed by Suzanne Somers. It is mostly fructose, so it should be used only in tiny amounts on the hypoglycemic diet and not at all for the weight-loss diet.

Sugar Substitute Equivalents

(Sweetener packets are all equal to 2 teaspoons of sugar, and 1 gram of carb.)

Sugar	Splenda Granular Sugar Twin Equal Spoonful	Packets (all)	Sweet'N Low Liquid	Stevia	AcesulfameK (Sweet One, etc.)
1 tsp	1 tsp	½ packet	10 drops	1/16 tsp powder, 2–4 drops	¼ tsp
1 tbs	1 tbs	1½	30 drops	1/5 tsp, 6–9 drops	3/8 tsp
¼ cup	½ cup	6	1½ tsp	½ tsp powder, ½ tsp liquid	3 tsp
⅓ cup	⅓ cup	8	2 tsp	⅔ tsp powder, ⅔ tsp liquid	4 tsp
½ cup	½ cup	12	1 tbs	½ tsp powder, ½ tsp liquid	2 tbs
1 cup	1 cup	24	2 tbs	1 tsp powder, 1 tsp liquid	4 tbs (¼ cup)

- Don't cook with NutraSweet or Equal. Aspartame loses its flavor when it's heated.
- 1 Equal tablet = 1 tsp sugar, or 1 tsp Splenda
  Tablets and liquids are the only way to get 0 grams of carbohydrate.

- *Xylitol* can be ordered from 917-441-1038, or purchased on the Internet. This has a minty flavor, so it's not the best choice for all foods.
- *Sorbitol* is used in many sugar-free candies and baked goods. Watch for GI upset: Gas, bloating, and diarrhea are common if you overdo it.

Measurements

General
2 tablespoons = 1 fluid ounce = ⅛ cup
3 teaspoons = 1 tablespoon
4 tablespoons = 2 fluid ounces = ¼ cup = 12 teaspoons
5⅓ tablespoons = ⅓ cup (5 tablespoons plus 1 teaspoon)
8 tablespoons = 4 fluid ounces = ½ cup = 24 teaspoons
1 cup = 8 fluid ounces = ½ pint = 240 milliliters = 16 tablespoons = 48 teaspoons
2 cups = 1 pint = 16 ounces
4 cups = 2 pints = 1 quart = 32 ounces
8 ounces = ½ pound
16 ounces = 1 pound
16 cups = 4 quarts = 1 gallon = 128 ounces

Butter
1 stick = 8 tablespoons = ½ cup = 4 ounces
4 sticks = 2 cups = 1 pound

Cheese
4 cups shredded = 1 pound = 16 ounces
2 cups cottage cheese = 1 pound = 16 ounces
1 cup cream cheese = 8 ounces
1 ounce cream cheese = 2 tablespoons
1 package cream cheese = 3 ounces = 6 tablespoons

Nuts
1 pound nuts = 3½ cups nuts (usually)
½ pound nuts = 1 cup chopped nuts

Can sizes
8-ounce can is about 1 cup

Chocolate
1 square = 1 ounce

Lemon/lime juice
1 lemon or lime yields 3–4 tablespoons juice

SOME OTHER LOW-CARB DIETS

As we've already said, there are many low-carbohydrate diet books on the market these days. Some contain recipes that are acceptable for our diets, especially the weight-loss diet, since they were all designed for that purpose. Use with caution, especially if you are carbohydrate sensitive or hypoglycemic, and always check each recipe for forbidden ingredients. This includes things like chocolate because of the caffeine content. One ounce should be your limit.

Dr. Atkins' New Diet Revolution: The late Dr. Robert C. Atkins, who was a cardiologist and the spokesman for the low-carb diet, began this program many years ago. He was subjected to much abuse for his trouble, but certainly gave as good as he got! He published many books, all of which are good resources. His sugar-free products are expensive but useful. This weight-loss diet has an induction phase that limits quantities of vegetables. This is stricter than some of the other weight-loss diets. His newer books have some more complicated concepts, but all are interesting.

Dr. Bernstein's Diabetes Solution: Today this approach seems radical, but as our chapter 6 on diabetes states, this was once the standard treatment for diabetes: restricting carbohydrates to control blood sugar. This book includes a section of recipes that are acceptable for the hypoglycemic diet but not for weight loss, because many use sugar-free flatbreads. This should be the textbook for diabetics and their families.

The Carbohydrate Addict's Diet: This diet was designed by two Ph.Ds, and basically allows no carbohydrates by day, but anything you want in the evening in a reward meal. The no-carb recipes are acceptable, but this premise is a disaster for hypoglycemics and those who are carbohydrate sensitive. Weight loss is, of course, much slower on this program even if you can manage to be successful on it.

Fran McCullough's *The Low-Carb Cookbook* and *Living Low-Carb* both have excellent recipes—not all of which are acceptable on our diets, because she allows some sugar and starch as well as caffeine. Excellent material and resource sections.

The Glucose Revolution: This diet book is based on the glycemic index of food. It forbids foods that may be particularly troublesome to carbohydrate-intolerant people. It has some limitations and flaws as far as most experts are concerned. Few of the recipes are acceptable for use with our diets.

Protein Power: This low-carb program was developed by medical doctors and includes recipe sections. This diet allows caffeine and other foods that hypoglycemics can't tolerate. It's too liberal for many to lose weight on, but most can maintain weight on this program. It requires a fair amount of calculation and counting of proteins and fats, allowing about thirty grams of carbohydrate a day.

The Paleolithic Prescription, The Stone Age Diet, **and** *Ne-anderthin:* The premise of this diet is to eat only what Stone Age folks did. It is very restrictive compared with more modern diets! The fruit allowance on some of these will not work for hypoglycemics.

Sugar Busters: This program mostly limits refined sugars. It allows many more carbs than other diets. A very few recipes are acceptable for our diets. This diet was designed by medical doctors. Portion control is necessary, unlike most other low-carbohydrate diets.

Suzanne Somers: Suzanne's books (*Get Skinny on Fabulous Foods, Eat Great Lose Weight,* and *Eat, Cheat, and Melt the Fat Away*) include some very good recipes, many of which can be used on our diets. This diet is complicated (food combining) and uses low-fat and whole wheat products, unlike most other low-carb diets. It's similar to the Montignac Diet—a French GI diet. Suzanne is now marketing diet products as well.

The Zone: Barry Sears's program is not strictly low carb, but does have some recipes that we can use. Most people can maintain weight on this program, but it may be too liberal for some who are sensitive to carbohydrates. It requires a lot of counting and measuring, and portion control.

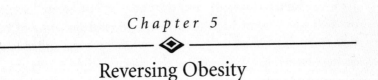

Chapter 5

Reversing Obesity

Weight loss . . . I lost sixty pounds. The low-carbohydrate diet works; you simply have to adhere to it. No cheats. None. Rocks are hard, water is wet, and things fall down. Do it. You'll feel great!

—Gwen W., Santa Monica, California

While we've had a great deal of success with patients who diligently take up the challenge to battle obesity, it is our mission to convince them of the benefits. For someone who doesn't feel well and lacks energy, foods often become a great source of comfort. If a patient has hypoglycemia, the propensity for obesity increases significantly. Our goal is always to encourage our patients and motivate them with the promise of increased energy and stamina.

With newer patients, it can be more of a challenge. When we've gone through the initial session with patients, we know what they'll have to endure to get well. It will take some intense cycles of pain and fatigue, and they may be just barely hanging on as it is. It seems hard to wish the reversal on some of our sicker patients. Then we pity those who've got the added curse of hypoglycemia. We consider the dietary adjustments they'll have to make, added to the fact that they'll have to work through the task of avoiding salicylates. When we're eye to eye with a visibly obese individual it's even more heartrending. The poor patient looks so exhilarated having just learned there is a good reason for his or her fatigue and assorted symptoms. But as medical professionals, we're not equally relieved. We fully realize the limited recovery potential and wonder if the patient suspects. If patients comply with what we ask, hypoglycemia vanishes swiftly, while fibromyalgia does its roller-coaster act and eventually stops. It's possible that both will clear completely in the end. But what about the drag on patients' energy level just towing those extra pounds? What about the damage that's being done to the overstressed joints, the blood vessels, and the entire circulatory system? Obesity causes fatigue, but it also causes damage that can't be repaired, unlike the other conditions we've discussed so far. Simply put, if you are severely overweight, you *will* have less energy. If you are overweight *and* fibromyalgic, you will be even more fatigued. It's as simple as that: The excess weight will contribute to your lack of energy.

It hardly seems necessary to describe obesity. The perception is immediate and the subject distasteful. No one wants to be overweight, much less obese. It's hard for physicians and hard for patients. Physicians know that whatever treatments they offer will be only partially successful: Patients will not be energized and complaint-free unless they can lose weight. Patients know that their physician is going to bring up the subject eventually, even if they just come around every once in a while with an unrelated complaint.

Obesity maims. Doctors call this morbidity. The initial five pounds seem innocuous enough, but the problem is that those few too often give way to the next fifty. Excess weight invites inertia, an ultimate thief of mobility. Eventually weight alone efficiently imposes physical restrictions on performance and promotes further disabilities. This combination gets added into our biologic calculators with two negative signs. The distance from the parking lot to the store becomes painful, especially when combined with the poor stamina and overwhelming fatigue of fibromyalgia. There's one main refuge—get to the biggest and softest chair. That's real solace from fatigue, even though it adds to the sentence hovering over the already imprisoned muscles and skeleton.

Obesity also kills. It may do so only in the long term, but most of us want to be around for quite a while. Fatness creates indolence and progressive inactivity. There's the stealthy approach of arthritis, which comes sooner and is more painful when excess weight is put into the equation. Cholesterol and other lipid cohorts become well-directed missiles aimed at arteries. Joined by hypertension and, almost inevitably, insulin resistance, the evil design is soon completed. This conglomeration has been labeled Syndrome X (metabolic syndrome); we'll visit it in chapter 6, on diabetes.

We won't attempt to identify the fine line that distinguishes overweight from obesity. What's the difference? In metabolic terms, both are dangerous, and both will sap your energy, although of course it's a matter of degrees. It's best to treat all excess weight as an enemy, and not spend time splitting hairs.

YOU ARE NOT ALONE

I was still more fibrofogged than I thought I should be. Many of you responded to me, try the diet! A couple of you challenged me, what did I have to lose? A couple of weeks of eating differently? One of you challenged me to one day; if I survived that, then the next day, et cetera. Thank you so very much. I've now lost thirty-seven pounds at sixteen weeks, two or three inches in the most significant places, and feel terrific! Have energy I don't know what to do with. I'm finally able to do some walking, which in turn helps with the energy. I still have forty more pounds to go, but I plan on being strict for six more months. I am a walking billboard for the diet.

—*Betty H.*

Recent statistics attest to the horrible epidemic of obesity in the American population. Using twenty-five pounds as a measure of excess, an increase of 5.5 percent occurred in just one year, between 1998 and 1999. That may not sound too startling, but since 1991, 57 percent of the population has fallen into this category. America and the rest of the affluent world are fattening up. In women of certain ethnic groups, the number rises as high as 74 percent. Excess weight is considered by some as the most common and dangerous pediatric problem in the United States. Nearly 25 percent of children are now considered obese. These facts put heavy people in the majority. Several clothing manufacturers have announced that their latest fashions will now include women's dress sizes sixteen to twenty-six. Little wonder our current secretary of health has declared a state of war on obesity.

Most of our fibromyalgic patients and many hypoglycemics have gained at least some weight in the course of their illness. When we compiled statistics on more than two thousand patients, we found that 36 percent of our fibromyalgic patients are overweight, defined as a gain of twenty or more pounds since the onset of their illness. The *average* gain is much greater, however: about *forty-seven pounds* per individual. Our hypoglycemic patients are slightly worse off. Using the same criteria, 40 percent are likely to be overweight.

If you asked your friends to write down their anonymous impressions of your frame, you would find very little discrepancy. The eyes of the beholder are pretty reliable gauges when deciding who is normal or overweight. We just don't allow ourselves to see us as others do. A single glance is usually enough to estimate what's too heavy for a particular body frame. Fine-tailored measurements have been devised but add little beyond what our eyes can easily perceive. Of course, we appear more scientific if we use calipers to determine skin thickness or make erudite calculations of the body mass index. Both are relevant determinations if we contemplate future comparisons or we're doing detailed research papers on the subject. For purposes of this book, however, we readily accept the man on the street's descriptive words *chubby, overweight, heavy,* or *really fat* as reasonably accurate estimates.

For purposes of our discussion and euphemisms aside, let's simply accept that any significant amount of excessive fat is obesity. Many people prefer numerical definitions, so let's agree that obesity begins when we get twenty to thirty pounds beyond our ideal weight.

IT'S A BIG PROBLEM

> When I first found the high-protein diets, I knew I was
> on the right track for the first time in my life because
> everything leveled off and I had more energy than I ever
> imagined. But many of those first diets were flawed, and
> carbohydrates are addictive, at least for me. For the first
> four months before my wedding I was absolutely strict,
> and I mean I ate *nothing* that I wasn't supposed to eat.
> During that time almost all of my fibro symptoms went
> away and I lost fifty pounds. Had I stayed on it after the
> wedding I would not be as bad as I am now, I'm sure. I
> "found" most of those lost pounds again, and my fibro-
> myalgia is back in full force.
>
> —*Phyllis, North Carolina*

Over the years, we've met two kinds of patients who are quite
insensitive to the fact that they need to diet. The first group is
in absolute denial. They earnestly believe every word they
utter when describing their meals, bite by bite. Quite often
there'll be a friend or family member sitting in a corner chair
of our examining room. During chance eye encounters, we
sometimes catch a sudden arch of an eyebrow that questions a
less-than-inclusive recitation. Most of the time the visitors
choose not to alienate their chubby companions by verbally
challenging the false declarations. It's our experience that if you
can't be honest about what you are eating, you won't get much
help from this chapter.

Other patients are fully aware that they never have and won't
now follow any outlined diet. They are marvelously honest and
candid about the fact that they have no intention whatsoever to

deprive themselves of any culinary treats. Obesity is one spoke of the energy wheel they will never repair. They're going to remain at least partial energy cripples—but perhaps the rest of this book will still offer other considerations for improvement.

Let's now get down to the business at hand. Among you are some significantly overweight individuals who got there with the help of some as-yet-unidentified genetic quirks. You eat, and your body seemingly converts everything to fat. It's as though your entire body is just a big storage warehouse. Your physiology is such that even when you seriously reduce calories, your cells retaliate and refuse to cooperate. They simply retrench and burn fewer calories. Your chubby parts continue to spread no matter how often you think lean, no matter how carefully you restrict your portions. Even your attempts at exercise add weight, since muscle bulking comes from protein, and that's heavier than fat. It's primarily for you that we write and dedicate this chapter.

Dieticians aren't alone when they flat-out say, "There's only one way to gain weight and that's to eat more calories than you can burn." Alternatively stated, you're taking in more energy from food than you're expending. Succinctly and tersely, we could also rephrase it less politely: *Your appetite is just too big for your metabolic needs.* But is this really true?

SO WHAT DO YOU DO?

I needed to lose about thirty pounds, but I was about to give up thinking the strict diet was impossible for me. Every time I tried it, I had a lot of trouble with cravings and extreme hunger that bordered on panic. Then someone suggested that I stick with it for at least four days, and the desperate hunger pains would disappear. I was skeptical but I hung in there and lo and behold it was true. All of a sudden I felt full on very little food; sometimes I had to remind myself to eat! In a month I lost fourteen pounds . . . some of that was probably water, as the weight loss has since slowed down. But I'm completely convinced it works, and I no longer have that exhausted feeling after I eat. I also find that yoga is a wonderful gentle activity to do in combination with the diet. I believe it helps with the weight loss and it's a fantastic pain reliever for the sore muscles of fibromyalgia.

—*Naomi J., Toronto, Ontario, Canada*

What *are* you supposed to do if you've already cut calories to starvation levels and haven't lost much of anything? Perhaps you feel as if you've even added a few pounds just looking at the forbidden foods that will have to be stricken from your list. You're afraid you'll be fat forever unless you do a forty-day fast and jog at least ten miles a day. Please cheer up. If this were true, why would we bother writing? If we didn't have a better idea than that, we certainly wouldn't be writing this book. This book is designed for those who can help themselves shift from idle into energy drive. Obviously we have a plan.

Pay attention to the people in your life—friends and especially family members. You'll observe almost universal eating habits. Do you notice a singular pattern that typifies the heavy ones? Watch for the I-love-my-bread, what's-a-meal-without-potatoes prevalence. See them wistfully linger their eyes on the pasta-laden menu and, ignoring all other listings, yield to temptation. For most, it's the little-bite-won't-hurt-you, or it's-a-special-occasion mentality that sinks them. You may well be in their numbers. Your willpower doesn't match the level of

starvation it would take to shed even a few pounds. Your resolve just hasn't improved with time, has it? Isn't there some
way to get back on track and lose weight?

RETHINKING THE WAY YOU EAT

My husband is diabetic, and I have fibromyalgia. We tried
the Atkins diet once but couldn't seem to stay on it. Then
I discovered that you need three things on your plate. So replace the once served "potatoes, rice, or pasta" with another
low-carbohydrate green vegetable—asparagus and spinach,
or broccoli and spinach, or asparagus and cabbage. Having
the three things on our plates made all the difference in the
world. Also, having dessert made up in the fridge for an
evening snack made all the difference in the world, and
keeps you from wanting the "old ice cream" treat. I have
custard cups made with cream and Splenda made up at all
times. Sometimes I serve the custard with strawberries,
sometimes just sprinkled with nutmeg. It is so delicious; we
both love it and never think of ice cream anymore.

With these methods we have been able to stay on the
diet for two months now. I have lost fifteen pounds and
my husband has lost seventeen, and we both feel so much
better. His blood sugar is under control, and I don't have
the highs and lows I used to have. Try it, it works.

—*Julia T., Globe, Arizona*

We're now at the heart of the matter, and from here on out it
may not be much fun. There's no way to get around the fact
that you must have gotten into this fix pretty much by eating
just as you're still doing. Look closely at your habits and don't

damn the fats and the proteins as the likely suspects. If you've tried cutting them out, you already know that this method didn't get you thin. It's no use blaming your inherited legacy, because that remains with you no matter what you do. It's time for realistic introspection that should lead to only one logical conclusion: *The foods you've eaten to get you fat are the very ones you must quit to make you lean.*

Your energy wheel has a spoke out of kilter: Its size is the impediment and adversely impacts the entire alignment. You'll need to get a smoother and stronger spin on the problem. You need some help to figure out what to do next.

Let's quickly review something we discussed in chapter 3, on hypoglycemia. You probably recall that it's mainly sugars and starches that stimulate the release of the hormone insulin. Carbohydrates are far more effective at doing this than protein and certainly fats. Since only insulin, our storage hormone, can put fat into fat cells, doesn't it make sense to avoid arousing its release so often and in such copious amounts?

We all know and envy people who eat anything and everything they relish. Lucky them—they just don't gain weight. But if you've read this far into this chapter, you already know, and we don't have to tell you, that you are not like that. For you it's as though a simple whiff of boiling pasta is sufficient to put a shaft of spaghetti directly into the next available fat cell; barely brushing against the pastry cart in a restaurant will expand your thighs. This hardly exaggerates the way you feel. And the sad truth is, until some Nobel Prize–earning discovery surfaces, this unjust sensitivity to carbohydrates will prevail. Judging by statistics, most of us have no choice but to avoid or carefully ration carbohydrates. They're the real enemy when it comes to controlling your weight.

You'd probably rather go to the torture rack than contemplate another diet. We'll understand if we have to take you there kicking and screaming. But take you there we must, and there are rewards. If you're willing to listen, and to work with what we want to teach you here, you can lose the weight you want to. You can do it without starvation, and without frustration, once you get the ball rolling. Your energy will improve, and so will your mood. Once you achieve your targeted weight, you may start cheating, but this time only with judicious restraint. The last lesson you'll need to learn is to back off well before the pounds pile back on.

We advocate a strict low-carbohydrate diet. This is an all-or-nothing program that permits no deviations. You'll immediately notice it's a calorie-laden diet. That's of no consequence, since you won't be releasing enough insulin to store fat. Banning carbohydrates gives the body no choice but to rely on fats for energy. Your body will use up its stored fat, and you'll lose inches right where you need to. The greater protein content of this diet protects against muscle loss and amply supplies the essential amino acids needed to sustain tissue building and repair. Happily, there are very few restrictions on quantity. You never go hungry since you can eat whenever you want. When you learn to avoid releasing squirts of insulin, you have nothing to fear.

We remind you again that *there are no essential carbohydrates*. The body easily manufactures whichever of those it needs, so avoiding them poses no threat to your health. Our weight-loss diet includes many so-called 5 percent vegetables. That's a simple numerical reference to the relatively small amount of carbohydrate they contain. As an added benefit, they're like a Who's Who in the nutrition hierarchy because of their high mineral and vitamin content. The liberal meat and dairy allowance further provides some of those nutritive provisions and plenty of fatty acids for energy production.

Some of you will be shaken by the serious contradictions we pose to some widely propagandized guidelines on nutrition. Not enough people have questioned the wisdom of low-fat and high-complex-carbohydrate diets. You've probably already done this and regularly insisted on low-fat or fat-free everything—and failed to impress your scale by one ounce. Worse yet, adhering to such dictates may have made you fatter than ever. If you're terribly uneasy about giving up most fruits and certain vegetables, strike a compromise with yourself. Though hardly necessary since the diet is self-contained, placate your conscience by adding one B-complex vitamin and a few calcium tablets daily. This is a diet to lose weight. If done right, you won't need to follow it forever.

There are just a few important things to remember when you read the diet that follows. The first cheerful fact is that unless specified, there is no limit to the amount you can eat from the list. You won't have to go hungry—but you can't cheat or you'll gain weight very quickly. Adding carbohydrates to this high-calorie diet is a recipe for disaster. You must follow instructions as they're written or you won't lose weight. Unlike a low-calorie diet, you can't substitute or swap foods around at your whimsy. All carbohydrates just aren't created equal.

The basic diet follows. Before beginning any new diet regimen, of course, you should consult your doctor or health-care practitioner. Notice how this differs from the more liberal diet we offered for hypoglycemia. We include sample recipes and a few ideas to get you on your way. We've both followed this diet and we've lost weight doing it. We know you can, too, and we'll help you.

LOW-CARB DIET FOR WEIGHT LOSS

MEATS All meats are allowed, except cold cuts that contain sugar. (*Check labels carefully. In particular, low-fat or nonfat turkey cold cuts usually have added dextrose or corn syrup.*) Bacon and ham are acceptable although they list sugar on the labels. The sugar cooks off and isn't a problem. Very heavy coatings are sometimes painted onto ham, and those should be scraped off. All fowl and game, fish and shellfish are allowed in unlimited quantities.

DAIRY PRODUCTS
Eggs
Any natural cheese (natural cheese is any cheese you slice yourself)
Cream (heavy and sour)
Cottage and whole-milk ricotta cheese (½-cup limit)
Butter and margarine

FRUITS
Fresh coconut
Avocado (limit ½ avocado per day)
Cantaloupe (limit ¼ melon per day)
Strawberries (limit 6–8 per day)
Lime or lemon juice (limit 2 teaspoons per day), for flavoring

VEGETABLES

Asparagus	Cabbage (limit 1 cup per day)
Bean sprouts	Cauliflower
Broccoli	Celery
Brussels sprouts	Chard

Chicory

Chinese cabbage (limit 2
  cups per day)

Chives

Cucumber

Daikon (long, white radish)

Eggplant

Endive

Escarole

Fennel

Garlic

Greens (mustard, beet)

Jicama

Kale

Leeks

Lettuce

Mushrooms

Okra

Olives

Parsley

Peppers (red, green, yellow, etc.)

Pickles (dill, sour; limit 1 per day)

Pimiento

Radicchio

Radish

Rhubarb

Salad greens

Sauerkraut

Scallions (green onions)

Spinach

String beans (green or yellow)

Snow peas

Summer squash (crookneck
  yellow or green)

Tomatoes

Water chestnuts

Watercress

Zucchini

NUTS (limit 12 per day)

Almonds

Brazil nuts

Butternuts

Filberts

Hazelnuts

Hickory nuts

Macadamia nuts

Pecans

Pine nuts (small handful)

Pistachios

Sunflower seeds (small handful)

Walnuts

DESSERTS
Sugar-free Jell-O
Custard (made with cream and artificial sweetener)
Cheesecake (no crust or nut crust with cream cheese, sour cream, and artificial sweeteners)

BEVERAGES
Artificially sweetened drink mixes like Crystal Light, Country Time, etc.
Diet sodas or mineral water with zero carbohydrates
Tea (unsweetened or made with sugar substitutes)
Coffee or decaffeinated coffee
Bourbon, cognac, gin, rum, Scotch, vodka, dry wine

*Important note: If you are overweight and hypoglycemic you must avoid all sources of caffeine.

CONDIMENTS AND SPICES
All spices including seeds (fresh or dried)
All imitation flavorings
Horseradish
Sugar-free sauces such as hollandaise, mayonnaise, mustard, ketchup, soy sauce, Worcestershire sauce
Sugar-free salad dressings
Oil and vinegar (all types)

MISCELLANEOUS
All fats
Caviar

*If cholesterol is a problem, avoid cold cuts except sugar-free turkey. Trim all visible fat off meat. Remove the skin from poultry. Broil or grill foods instead of frying. Avoid full-fat cheese, heavy cream, solid margarine, hollandaise sauce, and macadamia nuts. Use egg whites or Egg Beaters instead of whole eggs. Use liquid margarine only. Nuts should be dry-roasted only. Use canola or olive oil.

FOODS TO STRICTLY AVOID

These are the foods that you must absolutely avoid to lose weight:

Sweet wine, fruit brandy, and champagne
Baked beans, refried beans, black-eyed peas, kidney beans, lima beans
Bananas
Potatoes, corn, rice, barley, and pasta of any kind
Tamales, burritos, and flour tortillas
Dried fruits, fruit juices
Dextrose, glucose, hexitol, maltose, sucrose, honey, fructose, corn or cane syrup, or starch
Caffeine, if you are hypoglycemic

TWO-WEEK MEAL PLAN FOR WEIGHT LOSS

Here is a sample two-week menu for our weight-loss diet. We didn't use leftovers—something you'd do in real life, of course. We didn't here just to include more ideas for meals. Usually a breakfast casserole, a batch of egg custard, or a quiche will last for a few days.

We've also allowed two snack ideas a day, knowing full well

that most people on the diet won't eat that much. You can always use one of the snacks for an after-dinner treat if you're more of an evening eater than a morning eater. Not everyone will want a full breakfast. If you're not a breakfast person, feel free to skip it, and have a midmorning snack only if you like.

We didn't include beverages in the meal plans. You can add what you like from the diet, and in the quantity you prefer.

DAY 1

Breakfast	Sausage muffins
Snack	1 cup sugar-free Jell-O
Lunch	2 hot dogs with melted Jack cheese, sliced tomatoes, ½ cup cottage cheese
Snack	12 macadamia nuts, faux root beer float
Dinner	Chicken tenders, lemon spinach salad, roasted tomatoes

DAY 2

Breakfast	2 scrambled eggs with ½ cup ricotta cheese or any cheese, 6 strawberries
Snack	Low-carb protein bar
Lunch	Chef's salad
Snack	2 stalks of celery filled with cream cheese and 12 walnuts
Dinner	Sausage and peppers with zucchini fettuccine Parmesan

DAY 3

Breakfast Panna cotta
Snack   Protein shake
Lunch   Ham steak with green bean salad (or soup) and ½ cup cottage cheese
Snack   String or Jack cheese with 12 nuts
Dinner   Bacon-wrapped shrimp and cheese-covered mixed vegetables

DAY 4

Breakfast Protein shake
Snack   ¼ cantaloupe and ½ cup cottage cheese
Lunch   Egg salad lettuce rolls with sliced tomatoes and feta cheese
Snack   Sugar free Jell-O with sour cream topping
Dinner   Pork piccata with green beans amadine and caprese

DAY 5

Breakfast 2 fried eggs with ham and ½ cup cottage cheese
Snack   Chocolate mousse
Lunch   Roast beef rolls with cream cheese, horseradish, and shredded lettuce
Snack   Cucumber with walnuts and sour cream
Dinner   Pot roast with brussels sprouts, leeks, and horse-radish sauce

DAY 6

Breakfast Ham and cheese omelet with broiled tomato
Snack   English toffee and chocolate mousse
Lunch   Curried chicken salad
Snack   Cheese crisps
Dinner   Dilled salmon, faux tatoes, cucumbers and sour cream

DAY 7

Breakfast Protein shake with ¼ cantaloupe
Snack   Egg salad with cucumber chips and dill
Lunch   Cheese soufflé with tossed salad
Snack   Diet chocolate soda with whipped cream (float)
Dinner   Chicken with roasted asparagus and nutmeg summer squash

DAY 8

Breakfast Scrambled eggs, bacon, and broiled tomatoes with Parmesan cheese
Snack   Cantaloupe cubes and vanilla sour cream
Lunch   Caesar salad with chicken breast or shrimp
Snack   Pepperoni chips and Pepper Jack cheese
Dinner   Steak with bacon-stuffed mushroom caps and garlic vegetable puree

DAY 9

Breakfast Ham and cheese quiche

Snack	Strawberries or cantaloupe with crème fraiche
Lunch	Hot spinach salad with bacon
Snack	Diet cream soda float
Dinner	Scampi with baked spinach casserole

DAY 10

Breakfast	Spinach and Jack cheese omelet
Snack	Sugar-free Jell-O with cantaloupe or strawberries
Lunch	Chopped salad
Snack	Basil-wrapped hot dogs
Dinner	Stir-fried beef and faux fried rice

DAY 11

Breakfast	Egg custard and 6 strawberries
Snack	Sugar-free Jell-O
Lunch	Salade Niçoise Greek style
Snack	Pork rinds and sour cream or sugar-free salsa
Dinner	Maple pork tenderloin, roasted fennel, and herbed snow peas

DAY 12

Breakfast	Zucchini pancakes and sausage
Snack	¼ cantaloupe with squeezed lemon
Lunch	Tuna salad roll-ups
Snack	½ cup cottage cheese with 12 walnuts
Dinner	Pesto snapper and vegetables

DAY 13

Breakfast	Vanilla mousse with cantaloupe cubes
Snack	Sugar-free Jell-O with walnuts
Lunch	Avocado cheeseburger with salad
Snack	Deviled eggs
Dinner	Slow-cooker jambalaya and Gorgonzola faux tatoes

DAY 14

Breakfast	Sausage and egg cups
Snack	Protein shake with macadamia nuts
Lunch	Shrimp foo yung
Snack	Celery with Pepper Jack cubes
Dinner	Maple-glazed pork with faux fries and broccoli

SHOPPING LIST

This list is a basic list of ingredients you'll need for this menu plan. Quantities are not specified because appetites vary, and so will the number of people for whom you're cooking. For certain meals, choices have been offered, and you may want to make substitutions based on your own personal likes. For example, chicken stir-fry could be made with beef, pork, or shrimp. Use this list as a guide as you read through the recipes and make your choices.

Meat

Hot dogs (kosher are sugar-free)—1 package
1 small precooked ham (probably the best way to provide for the recipes here)

Sliced roast beef (2–3 slices per person; slightly more if using in chef's or chopped salad)
Chicken breasts (or thighs if preferred), boneless
Large bag precooked large shrimp
Chuck roast
Steaks (boneless, for 1 dinner and stir-fry)
Hamburger meat
Spareribs (1 meal)
Pork chops (boneless) and 1 pork loin, or 1 large loin for 2 meals
Salmon steaks
Red snapper fillets
Bacon
Pepperoni
Salami
Sugar-free Italian sausage
Sugar-free breakfast sausage
3 cans of tuna

Eggs and/or Egg Beaters if preferred

Dairy
Cottage cheese (large container)
Sour cream (large container)
Cream cheese (large container)
Whipping cream (get a big one)
Jack cheese, or Pepper Jack if preferred
Cheddar cheese
Swiss cheese
String cheese (if preferred for snacks)
Crumbled feta cheese (for salad)

Gorgonzola cheese
Parmesan cheese
Small container full-fat ricotta
Butter

Vegetables
Spinach (washed bag, for salads)
Spinach (frozen, for omelet)
Lettuce (for salads and roll-ups)
Celery stalks
Green beans—cans for soup/lunch salad
Zucchini (at least 10)
Yellow crookneck (summer) squash
Bean sprouts
Jicama
Avocado (1)
Scallions (for salads)
Fresh or Frozen (buy amounts according to preferences):
  Broccoli
  Brussels sprouts
  Cauliflower
  Celery root
  Green beans
Snow peas

Herbs and Spices
Garlic
Fresh dill
Horseradish—bottled is easiest
Ginger (fresh or grated)
Fresh basil leaves

Ground cumin
Chili pepper
Crushed red pepper flakes
Onion powder
Garlic salt
Nutmeg
Rosemary
Caraway seeds
Celery seeds
Vanilla extract

Nuts
Macadamia nuts (large bag)
Walnuts, pecans, or whichever nut you prefer from diet list for snacks
Almonds (slivered, 1 bag)

Miscellaneous
Capers
Coconut milk (unsweetened)
Dijon mustard
Gelatin (unflavored)
Greek olives
Jalapeño peppers (if you like hot peppers)
Lemon juice (or fresh lemons for juice)
Maple syrup (sugar-free)
Olive oil
Peanut oil
Pesto sauce (usually sugar-free, but check)
Pork rinds (these are pure protein and can be used as breading, or as crunchy snacks)

Soy sauce (sugar-free)
Vinegar
White Worcestershire sauce
Wine for cooking: Red wine, white wine, marsala, or brandy
Wooden toothpicks

Diet Supplies
Protein powders: vanilla, chocolate, or other flavors
Low-carbohydrate diet protein bars
Splenda
Sugar-free mayonnaise
Sugar-free syrups (Da Vinci or Torani): vanilla, English toffee, caramel, etc.

RECIPES

DAY ONE

Sausage Muffins

You can make these the night before and reheat in microwave or oven. Preheat the oven to 375 degrees. Lightly brown 1 pound of sausage patties or sausage meat, and set aside. Grease a small muffin tin (4–6 muffins) or a small square baking pan. If you are using precooked sausage patties, just crumble—there is no need to heat them. Beat 4 eggs in a bowl, and add 1 cup of heavy cream, ½ teaspoon of salt, ½ teaspoon of pepper, and ½ cup of protein powder. Fold in ½ cup of grated Cheddar cheese and ½ cup of grated Swiss cheese. Gently stir in the sausage meat and pour into the muffin tins or baking dish. Bake for 15 minutes, until set and turning brown. Makes 4 to 6 muffins.

Faux Root Beer Float

Whip ⅓ cup of heavy cream and put in the bottom of a glass. Pour in diet root beer slowly. This will foam up and can be eaten with a spoon and sipped just like the real version.

Chicken Tenders

Preheat the oven to 350 degrees. Take boneless, skinless chicken breasts and pound them with a kitchen mallet to make them thin and flat. Cut into strips. Mix together 1 cup of mayonnaise (for 3 medium-size breasts) with 1 tablespoon of lemon juice and ½ teaspoon of garlic salt. (Optional: Add 1 teaspoon of dried herbs such as rosemary or tarragon.) Coat the chicken strips thickly and let sit for an hour at room temperature. Bake until golden brown, about 45 minutes. Turn once when the first side is brown. Serves 4.

Spinach Salad

Tear spinach into bite-size pieces, and put into a salad bowl. In a small bowl, mix ½ cup of olive oil and 2½ tablespoons of lemon juice. Whisk together until well mixed. Season with garlic salt to taste; the dressing should be a little tart. Pour on the spinach and toss well.

Roasted Tomatoes with Garlic

The oven is preheating for chicken—350 degrees. Cut tomatoes in half lengthwise. Coarsely chop 1 garlic clove for each tomato. Brush a cookie sheet with olive oil, and place the tomato halves on it, faceup. Sprinkle the garlic over the tomatoes, and put a tiny dab of olive oil on top. Bake for 45 minutes.

DAY TWO

Chef's Salad

Tear lettuce into bite-size pieces. Over the top, arrange sliced chicken or turkey, sliced ham, sliced cheese (Cheddar, Swiss, Jack, or a combination), and 2 hard-boiled eggs. Garnish with two slices of avocado, tomato, radishes, cucumbers, olives, and other vegetables.

Mustard Vinaigrette

In a blender combine ½ cup of olive oil, 2 tablespoons of red wine vinegar, 2 chopped garlic cloves, ½ teaspoon of Dijon mustard, a dash of white Worcestershire sauce, and salt and pepper to taste.

Sausage and Peppers

Use ¾ cup uncooked sliced peppers per sausage. Core peppers, removing the white core and ribs and rinsing away the seeds. Slice into long strips. Heat olive oil in a skillet over medium to medium-high heat and add the peppers. Season with garlic salt and cook until soft. Remove the peppers from the skillet and add sausage. If precooked, simply cook until brown. If uncooked, place ½ inch of water in the skillet with the sausages and cook until the water steams away. Then add a small amount of olive oil and fry the sausages until brown. When the sausages are cooked, add the peppers, stir together, and heat. Garnish with crushed red pepper if desired.

Zucchini Fettuccine Parmesan

Cut the ends off zucchini and peel. Continue with the vegetable peeler, making broad ribbons from the zucchini. Soak the zucchini ribbons for 15 minutes in water into which a lemon has been squeezed. Melt butter in a skillet (1 tablespoon for every 2 zucchini) with a clove of chopped garlic. Drain the zucchini and pat it dry in paper towels. Cook it in the skillet until it is the texture of cooked pasta. If necessary, drain off excess butter. Add Parmesan cheese and salt to taste. Toss and serve. You can also use summer squash for this dish, and add any herbs you like. Makes 2 large servings.

DAY THREE

Panna Cotta

Make this the night before. This wonderful Italian dish can also be eaten as a dessert or snack. You can serve it with any of the sugar-free syrups like raspberry, or with strawberries.

Place 4 tablespoons of warm water in a small bowl and sprinkle with a packet of unflavored gelatin. Let this sit for about 10 minutes. In a small saucepan, heat 1½ cups of heavy cream and 2 teaspoons of vanilla extract to a boil over medium heat. When this mixture comes to a boil, add the water and gelatin, and stir in another 1½ cups of heavy cream and ½ cup of Splenda. Pour the mixture right away into 6 custard cups or any small cups. Chill until cold and set, about 3 hours.

Green Bean Salad

Put 2 cans of green beans in the refrigerator the night before. To make the salad, open the cans and drain the green beans. Toss with 1 tablespoon white wine or balsamic vinegar and salt or garlic salt to taste. Serves 4 as a side dish.

Green Bean Soup

Drain 2 cans of green beans (but reserve the liquid) and put into the blender. Add 1½ cups of heavy cream and blend. Add the reserved liquid from the beans until soup is at the desired consistency. Add ⅛ teaspoon each of salt, cumin, and pepper. Add a dash of white Worcestershire sauce, if desired. Heat in the microwave or a saucepan. Serve with a dollop of sour cream, if desired. Makes 2 large servings.

Bacon-Wrapped Shrimp

Preheat the broiler. Use precooked shrimp; have them at room temperature. Use ½ slice of bacon for each shrimp. You can precook the bacon for a minute or two in the microwave if you like your bacon well done. If you like jalapeño peppers, place one on each shrimp. If you prefer cheese, use a crumbled piece of Jack, feta, or Gorgonzola. Wrap the bacon around the shrimp and filling, and secure with a wooden toothpick or skewer. Place on a cookie sheet and put under the broiler until the bacon is cooked and the cheese is melted.

Cheese-Covered Vegetables

Heat the broiler. Cut into large pieces a combination of zucchini, yellow squash, mushrooms, red pepper strips, broccoli, cauliflower—whatever you like. Use a vegetable steamer and pot, or steam in the microwave. Cook hard vegetables (broccoli, cauliflower, brussels sprouts) until partially soft, and then add softer ones such as green beans, pepper strips, mushrooms, and squash. When the vegetables are all slightly tender, transfer them into a wide baking dish. Top with slices of cheese of your choice. Place under the broiler and cook until the cheese is melted, bubbly, and starting to turn brown. Season with ground pepper or crushed red peppers.

DAY FOUR

Egg Salad Rolls

Chop the desired number of hard-boiled eggs with a fork. Add spoonfuls of sugar-free mayonnaise until the egg salad is the desired consistency. Slice a tomato. Take lettuce leaves and lay them flat. Spread egg salad along the leaf, and top with tomato slices. Add some chopped lettuce on top, and whatever else you'd like (bean sprouts, an avocado slice, chopped olives, a spoonful of capers). Fold the lettuce around the salad to form a pocket.

Pork Piccata

This recipe is for 4 boneless pork chops. Pound the chops with a kitchen mallet until they are about ¼ to ½ inch thick. If the pork chops are thick, butterfly them (slice in half the long way) first. Dust the chops with low-carb baking mix or protein powder. Heat 2 tablespoons of butter in a skillet until bubbly. Add the pork to the skillet and brown both sides. Remove and set aside. Add ½ cup of white wine, 2 tablespoons of lemon juice, and a tablespoon of capers to the skillet and cook over medium heat until the sauce is reduced. Add 4 tablespoons of butter as it cooks. Return the pork to the pan and re-heat with the sauce. Pour the sauce over the pork chops and serve. Serves 4.

Green Beans Amandine

Cook 2 cups of green beans in a microwave or on the stovetop. In a small frying pan, cook 2 tablespoons slivered almonds in butter until they are golden. Add ½ teaspoon of salt and 1 teaspoon of lemon juice. Add the green beans and toss until well mixed. Serves 2.

Caprese Salad

large beefsteak tomatoes, sliced
buffalo mozzarella or other soft mozzarella, sliced
chopped basil
olive oil

Slice the tomatoes and lay them flat on a plate. On top of each tomato slice, add a slice of mozzarella. Put fresh basil on top, and drizzle with olive oil.

DAY FIVE

Chocolate Mousse

Place 1 cup of whipping cream in a bowl. Add a scoop of chocolate protein powder and beat. Add more cream to taste, if desired. You can also add a dash of sugar-free syrup (chocolate hazelnut or chocolate raspberry mousse). Serves 2. (It is filling.)

Roast Beef Rolls

Put large lettuce leaves on a plate. Top each with a slice of roast beef. In a small bowl, put ½ cup of cream cheese. Add horseradish to taste, and mash together with a fork. Spread the mixture on the roast beef, and top with chopped lettuce. Fold the lettuce leaves in half to make a sandwich. Serves 2.

Cucumber with Walnuts and Sour Cream

In a small bowl, put ½ cup of sour cream. Coarsely chop 10 walnuts and add to the sour cream. Peel and slice a cucumber into cracker-size chips. Dip into the sour cream mixture and eat.

Pot Roast with Vegetables

Buy a pot roast, chuck roast, or seven-bone roast. Preheat the broiler. When it's hot, place the roast on an oven-safe dish or cookie sheet and place under the broiler to sear. When the meat is browned (about 10 minutes), remove and place in a large skillet. Fill the skillet about 1 inch deep with liquid. This can be water, red wine, bouillon, or a mixture of these. Cover tightly and cook for about 1½ hours, until it cuts deeply with a fork, adding more liquid if necessary. (You will want some pan liquid for gravy.) If you wish, add vegetables and cook for the last 20 minutes. If not, steam vegetables and serve on the side with pan juice. Wonderful with horseradish sauce. Serves 4 with leftovers.

To prepare vegetables:
Cut off the dark green portion of a leek, and peel away the outer leaves. Slice lengthwise, and steam. For brussels sprouts, peel off the dark green outer leaves if wilted.

Horseradish Sauce

Mix ½ cup of sour cream with ½ cup of heavy cream and ½ teaspoon of white Worcestershire sauce. Stir in 2–3 tablespoons of horseradish, or more to taste.

DAY SIX

English Toffee Chocolate Mousse

Make mousse as before (see day 5), adding English toffee syrup to the mixture.

Curried Chicken Salad

To 1 cup of chopped chicken, add ½ cup of chopped celery, 1 finely chopped scallion, and ¼ cup of chopped water chestnuts. (Add a small amount of chopped dill pickle, capers, or chopped olive if you like.) Mix together with ½ cup of sugar-free mayonnaise to which 2 tablespoons of curry powder has been added. Salt and pepper to taste. Serves 2.

Cheese Chips

Grate 1 cup of Cheddar cheese. Oil a skillet or griddle with a paper towel dipped into olive or cooking oil. Put lumps of cheese on the pan and fry until brown. Flip over and continue cooking for another minute. Drain on paper towels. You can crumble bacon into the cheese before cooking for a variation. Makes 8 to 10 chips.

Dilled Salmon

Preheat the oven to 400 degrees. Have a salmon fillet at room temperature. This sauce will work for about 2 pounds of fish. Mix 1 cup of sour cream, ½ cup of snipped fresh dill, 1 tablespoon of mustard, 2 chopped green onions, and 2 chopped garlic cloves in a bowl with salt and pepper to taste. Grease a baking dish or baking sheet with olive oil. Place the salmon on the dish skin down, and spread with a thick layer of the sour cream mixture (use about half). Bake until the salmon is pink—about 30 minutes. Serve with the remainder of the sauce. Serves 4.

Faux Tatoes

Peel 2 medium-size celery roots and chop them into large pieces. Steam in a pan or in the microwave until very soft, about 15 minutes, making sure the mix is mushy. Put the celery root in a blender or food processor and puree, adding 3 tablespoons of butter and ½ cup of cream until smooth and the consistency of mashed potatoes. Add salt and pepper to taste. Serves 2.

Cucumbers and Sour Cream

Peel and slice cucumber(s). For each cucumber mix together ½ cup of sour cream with 2 teaspoons of white vinegar. Add salt, pepper, and a dash of onion powder to taste. Toss the cucumbers into the dressing and coat well. Serves 2.

DAY SEVEN

Egg Salad with Dill

Mash hard-boiled eggs with a fork, and add sugar-free mayonnaise to taste. Also add 1 teaspoon of snipped dill for each egg. Eat with cucumber chips or celery stalks.

Cheese Soufflé

Preheat the oven to 425 degrees. Butter a 6-cup soufflé dish thoroughly. Beat 6 egg yolks with ½ teaspoon of cayenne pepper, a dash of salt, and a dash of pepper until fluffy. Fold in ½ cup of cream cheese (make sure it is at room temperature before you start to cook) and then ½ cup each of grated Swiss and Jack cheese. In a separate bowl or in a blender, whip 6 egg whites until they are very stiff and form peaks. Fold the whites into the egg yolk mixture very gently. Pour the mixture gently into the greased soufflé dish and bake for 10 minutes. Lower the oven temperature to 400 degrees and bake for 15 more minutes. Serve right away. Serves 6.

Roast Chicken

The oven is already hot for the soufflé and asparagus. Place a cut-up chicken in a glass baking dish. Dot each piece with a piece of butter, and sprinkle with garlic salt, paprika, and ground cumin. Put a dash of lemon on each piece. Place this dish under the broiler, and cook for about 30 minutes. Turn frequently. Serves 4.

Roasted Asparagus

The oven is already heated to 400 degrees for the soufflé. Cut the hard end of the stems off ½ pound of asparagus. Place in a glass baking dish with 1 tablespoon of olive oil, and salt and pepper to taste. (You can also use garlic salt.) Roll the asparagus around until it is completely coated, and in a single layer. Cover the baking dish with aluminum foil and bake for 10 minutes. Remove from the oven, stir the asparagus, and return the dish to the oven without the aluminum foil. Cook for another 10 minutes. Serves 4.

Philippe's Yellow Squash

Cut the ends off 5 yellow squash, and slice about ½ inch thick. In a skillet, heat 1 tablespoon of olive oil and 1 tablespoon of butter until bubbly. Add the squash and sauté until soft. Remove from the heat, sprinkle with nutmeg, and serve immediately. Serves 4.

DAY EIGHT

Vanilla Sour Cream

Add a splash of vanilla sugar-free syrup to sour cream and stir together. Other flavors such as caramel, English toffee, or gingerbread work as well.

Caesar Salad with Shrimp or Chicken Breast

Shred 4 cups of romaine lettuce. Bring a small pot of water to a boil and drop in an egg, letting it cook for 1 minute only. (Or skip this step and set aside 1 egg's worth of egg substitute.) Drop 1 minced garlic clove in a wooden salad bowl, and add ½ teaspoon of Dijon mustard and a dash of lemon juice, about ½ teaspoon or so. Add a dash of Worcestershire sauce and Tabasco, if desired. Mash these ingredients together with a small amount of anchovy paste, if you like anchovies. Then whisk in 2 tablespoons of olive oil, and break the egg into the mixture, continuing to whisk well. Add the lettuce to the bowl and toss, adding 2–3 tablespoons of Parmesan cheese depending on how dry you like your salad. Add a broiled chicken breast or some shrimp to the salad (hot or cold). Serves 2 as a main course.

Pepperoni Chips

Place pepperoni on a paper towel, and cover with another. Microwave until crisp, about a minute. Excellent with Pepper Jack or white Cheddar slices. Makes 4 servings.

Mushroom Caps

This recipe calls for ½ pound of mushrooms, but can be easily doubled. Preheat the oven to 350 degrees. After washing the mushrooms, remove the caps and set aside. Chop the stems finely and add ½ teaspoon of onion powder. Sauté in a small frying pan in 1 tablespoon of butter until soft; this will take a few minutes. Add ½ cup of walnuts and 1 tablespoon of pork rinds that have been ground in a blender. Season with 1½ teaspoons of lemon juice. Place the caps skin-side down in a baking dish and stuff with the mixture you've just made in the pan. Fill a ¼-cup measuring cup with half white wine and half cream. Mix and put one large spoonful over each inverted cap. Bake for 20 minutes.

Steak au Poivre

Crush 1 tablespoon of peppercorns with a rolling pin (put them inside a plastic bag), or use coarsely ground pepper. Put the peppercorns on a cutting board, and press steaks on top until well coated. Pan-fry the steaks in a heavy skillet with 1 tablespoon of olive oil for each steak (5 minutes a side will give you medium rare). Remove the steaks from the pan. Add ½ cup of heavy cream and 1 tablespoon of brandy to the skillet and heat to a boil, stirring and scraping the bottom of the pan as you go. Lower the heat and cook for about 3 minutes, until the sauce is thick. Pour over the steaks and serve.

Vegetable Puree with Garlic

Steam 2 heads of broccoli (or an equal amount of fennel, red peppers, or leeks) until soft in the microwave or in a pot. Combine with 4 garlic cloves, heavy cream, salt, and pepper in the blender or food processor. Puree for about 2 minutes, until smooth. Add butter, salt, and pepper to taste. Serves 4.

DAY NINE

Ham and Cheese Quiche

Preheat the oven to 350 degrees. Butter a quiche pan. Beat 6 eggs in a bowl with a cup of heavy cream, salt, and pepper. Add 1 cup of grated Swiss or Cheddar cheese and ½ cup of ham; mix together. Pour into a quiche pan and bake for 40 minutes. Serve hot or cold.

Crème Fraiche

Buy commercially or mix heavy cream and sour cream half and half and let sit overnight.

Spinach Salad with Bacon

Heat 1 tablespoon of olive oil in a skillet. Add 4 slices of bacon that have been cut into ½-inch pieces, and cook until browned. Add 2 tablespoons of chopped walnuts or pine nuts, and 2 chopped garlic cloves. Cook for a minute longer. Remove the skillet from the heat; add 6 cups of spinach and a tablespoon of wine or balsamic vinegar, and toss well before serving.

Shrimp Scampi

This recipe is for ½ pound of shelled shrimp. Preheat the oven to 350 degrees. In a glass baking dish, put ½ cup of butter and ½ cup of white wine with 3 tablespoons of chopped garlic. If you do not want to use wine, you can use chicken stock or water with a squeeze of lemon juice. Bake for 5 minutes, until the shrimp is pink. Serves 2.

Baked Spinach

The oven is already preheated to 350 degrees for shrimp. Combine 1 cup of whole-milk ricotta, a dash of salt and pepper, and ½ teaspoon of white Worcestershire sauce in a blender. Blend until smooth, adding 2 eggs as you go. Combine this mixture in a baking pan with a package (10 ounces) of chopped frozen spinach and 2 teaspoons of caraway seeds, and sprinkle ½ cup grated Jack (or Cheddar) cheese over the top. Bake for 25 minutes. Serves 4.

DAY TEN

Chopped Salad

Finely chop salad ingredients: tomato, cheese, lettuce, salami, ham or roast beef, chicken, cucumbers, black olives, yellow or red bell peppers, radishes, or what have you. You can use any combination you like. Chop everything very finely and toss together well.

Dressing

In a small bowl, whisk together ¼ cup of olive oil, 1 tablespoon of lemon juice, 1½ teaspoons of Splenda, 1 small minced garlic clove, ½ teaspoon of salt, and a dash of pepper. When completely mixed, pour over the salad and toss well.

Basil-Wrapped Hot Dogs

Cut hot dogs into 1-inch pieces. Wrap with a fresh basil leaf and microwave for 1 minute.

Stir-Fried Beef

For a pound of sliced sirloin beef: Heat ½ cup of peanut oil in a wok or large pan. Drop in 2 minced garlic cloves, 1 teaspoon of ginger, the meat, and 2 stalks of chopped celery. Cook for a few minutes and add other chopped vegetables: 1 can of sliced water chestnuts, red pimientos, bean sprouts, snow peas, broccoli florets, small mushrooms, shredded cabbage, or what have you. When this is nearly cooked, toss in 1 cup of sugar-free teriyaki sauce or soy sauce. Remove the meat and vegetables from the pan, leaving the cooking juices behind. Cook to reduce the sauce, and when it is about half the volume, remove the wok from the heat. Stir in ⅓ stick of cold butter and ⅛ teaspoon of cayenne pepper. Add the other ingredients back to the wok, toss, and serve. Seves 4.

Faux Fried Rice

Chop finely or grate 1½ cups of raw cauliflower and set aside. In a small bowl, chop 1 scallion finely (keeping the white and green parts separate), ½ cup of water chestnuts, 2 garlic cloves, and 3 green beans—these can be frozen. (The cauliflower and water chestnuts should be the size of rice grains, and the green beans should be the size of peas.) In a wok or a frying pan, heat 1 tablespoon of peanut oil. Fry the chopped garlic and white part of the scallions for about a minute, and then add the cauliflower and water chestnuts. Stir while cooking for about 4 minutes. Add 2 tablespoons of sugar-free soy sauce, ½ teaspoon of ginger, the green part of the scallions, and the green beans. Stir together while cooking. Make a bare spot in the middle of the pan, pour in 2 beaten eggs, and stir until the eggs are cooked and then mixed in well. (You may need to add a bit more oil before adding the eggs if the pan is dry and it looks like they will stick.) Season with ground pepper. Serves 4.

DAY ELEVEN

Egg Custard

Preheat the oven to 350 degrees. Beat together 1 egg and 1 egg yolk (or add an egg yolk to the proper amount of an egg substitute). Add ½ cup of heavy cream and ½ cup of water (at room temperature). Add 3 tablespoons of Splenda and 1 teaspoon of vanilla. Pour into 2 custard cups. Set the custard cups in a pot that is about an inch full of warm water, and carefully put this in the oven. Bake for 30 minutes. Sprinkle the tops with nutmeg. Serves 2.

Salade Niçoise

In a large wooden salad bowl, whisk together 3 tablespoons of olive oil and 1½ teaspoons of red wine or balsamic vinegar. Add 2 cans of tuna (in oil, but drained). Add 1 peeled and chopped cucumber, 1 chopped tomato, 6 chopped Greek olives, and ½ cup of chopped scallions. Mix together well, and put on a bed of shredded romaine lettuce. Sprinkle with feta cheese. Serves 2.

Maple Pork Tenderloin

This can be made in the oven or on the grill. For a 1-pound pork tenderloin, begin by seasoning the meat with salt and pepper. Then wrap 4 slices of bacon around the pork and secure in place with wooden toothpicks. Brush the pork with sugar-free maple syrup. For a grill, set on medium heat and cook for about 20 minutes, turning occasionally and basting with the maple syrup. In an oven, set the oven to 350 degrees and bake for about 45 minutes, basting with the maple syrup and turning twice. Serves 4.

Snow Peas with Herb Butter

Drop ½ pound of snow peas into a pot of boiling salted water. Cook for only about 2 minutes, until they turn brighter green. Drain well. Toss the peas with 1 tablespoon of butter, ½ teaspoon of lemon juice, and ½ teaspoon of tarragon. Salt and pepper to taste. Serves 4 as a side dish.

Roasted Fennel

After washing 1–2 stalks of fennel, cut off the ends, cutting down to where the flesh is tender. Slice into thick slices, about ½ inch thick. Heat 1 tablespoon of oil per stalk over medium heat. Add the fennel and cook until it is soft, stirring continuously. Add salt and pepper to taste. Sprinkle the fennel liberally with Parmesan, Romano, or any hard cheese, and place under the broiler until the cheese is puffy, bubbly, and starting to turn brown, about 5 minutes. Serves 4 as a side dish.

DAY TWELVE

Zucchini Pancakes

Grate coarsely about 4 cups of zucchini into a bowl. Add ½ teaspoon of salt, and toss together. Let the zucchini sit for at least 15 minutes. Remove the mixture from the bowl and squeeze out the liquid. Return to the bowl and stir in 2 beaten eggs, ½ cup of Parmesan cheese, and a dash of granulated garlic powder or 1 garlic clove, chopped. Make patties of the zucchini mixture. Melt the butter in the skillet and fry the pancakes until golden, about 5 minutes a side. (Add more butter as needed to the pan so the pancakes don't stick.) Serves 4 as a side dish.

Ham and Cheese Roll-Ups

Lay lettuce or cabbage leaves flat on a plate. Spread with sugar-free mayonnaise or Dijon mustard. Add ham, cheese, and tomato, if desired. Fold over the lettuce leaf.

Snapper with Vegetables and Pesto Sauce

Preheat the oven to 350 degrees. For 2 snapper fillets: Mix together $\frac{2}{3}$ cup of pesto with 2 tablespoons of lemon juice. Tear a sheet of aluminum foil for each piece of snapper (10 x 12 inches). Place the piece of fish in the center of the foil sheet. Spread the pesto mixture over the top of the snapper. Top this with mixed vegetables cut into bite-size pieces—asparagus, tomato, squash, broccoli—then top with a spoonful of the pesto mixture. Fold together the foil sheet, sealing well. Put the packets on a baking sheet and cook for 30 minutes. Serves 2.

DAY THIRTEEN

Vanilla Coconut Mousse

Add 1 cup whipping cream to 1 cup unsweetened coconut milk. Using a hand mixer, add 2 to 3 tablespoons of vanilla protein powder and mix until firm. Serves 2.

Deviled Eggs

Hard boil 4 eggs. Refrigerate overnight, then peel them and cut them in half the long way. Remove the yolks to a small bowl and mash with a fork. Add 1 tablespoon of sugar-free mayonnaise and $\frac{1}{2}$ teaspoon of sugar-free mustard. Mix together well, and spoon the yolk mixture back into the whites. Garnish with paprika or chopped parsley.

Crock-Pot Jambalaya

Slow cookers or Crock-Pots are wonderful for this diet. Inexpensive cuts of meat will be cooked until extremely tender, and your dinner can be ready when you get home! Many recipes work for these cookers, and for many others you can easily substitute permissible vegetables for starchier ones.

In a Crock-Pot, combine about 1 pound of boneless skinless chicken, 2 chopped green peppers, 3 chopped celery stalks, at least 4 chopped garlic cloves, ½ cup of sugar-free tomato paste, 1 can of beef broth, 1 teaspoon of cayenne pepper, 2 teaspoons of Tabasco, 1 pound of cut-up hot sausage, ½ teaspoon of oregano, 1 teaspoon of basil, ½ teaspoon of rosemary, 1 can of tomatoes (14 ounces), drained, and 2 chopped green peppers. Cook for 4 hours on high; in the last 30 minutes, add 1 pound of shrimp. Serves 4.

Blue Cheese Faux Tatoes

Steam 2 pounds of cauliflower until very soft, and put in the blender. Add ½ cup of heavy cream, ½ cup of Gorgonzola or blue cheese, and 1 cup of sugar-free mayonnaise. Mix until smooth. Sprinkle with crumbled cooked bacon if you wish. Serves 2.

DAY FOURTEEN

Shrimp Foo Yung

Chop ½ cup of celery and cook in the microwave for 1 minute, until soft but still crisp. In a bowl, mix together 2 cups of chopped bean sprouts with ¼ cup of chopped shrimp and 6 beaten eggs. Add the celery to this mixture. Put 2 tablespoons of peanut oil in a skillet with 1 teaspoon of ginger and heat until bubbly. Form 4 cakes of this mixture and place in hot oil. Cook until brown on both sides. Serve with sugar-free soy sauce. Serves 4.

French-Fried Zucchini

Peel zucchini and cut it into thin, long strips. Heat 3 inches of peanut oil in a skillet. When the oil is very hot, add the zucchini sticks. Turn them until they are brown all over, and remove from the pan. Drain on paper towels, salt them, and serve them.

Coleslaw

This recipe is for 2 servings. Only 1 cup of cabbage a day is allowed on the weight-loss diet. In a large bowl, combine 1 cup of sour cream, 4 tablespoons of water, 1 packet of Splenda, ½ teaspoon of onion powder, ½ teaspoon of celery seeds, and 2 teaspoons of apple cider vinegar. Toss in 2 cups of shredded cabbage, and coat well. Refrigerate for an hour before serving.

OBSTACLES YOU'LL HAVE TO HURDLE

The obesity picture looks bleak because it is. It's difficult to lose weight, and more difficult to keep it off. While we've known many overweight people aged seventy or eighty, few brag much about their level of activity, or the quality of their lives. They've usually managed to deal with their weight by progressively curtailing their activities. Sheepishly, these folks have given in to their status of quasi-invalidism. They steadfastly do a little less a lot slower, and will probably die a little faster.

There are many stumbling blocks to reconfiguring your

waistline, and you can certainly make them insurmountable because *you* are the worst of these. The obstacles are your bad habits. You may have to fight yourself daily. It's hard, we know, but you can do it. It's time to damn the excuses—full speed ahead! Only you can muster the willpower that has thus far eluded you. Luckily, the rewards are many, and they don't take long to reap, especially the exhilaration that will come from losing the weight that's been your enemy for so long.

As we've learned from Alcoholics Anonymous, you must first admit that you have a problem and you can't eat everything you want to. Acknowledge past limitations and failures. You've always capitulated to your weakness for certain foods. Similarly, you've easily surrendered when family and friends tempted you. Sadly, despite their reassurances, even a little bite *did* hurt you. It takes courage, and you must find that within yourself.

Restaurant and packaged food errors only *seem* beyond your control. That just isn't true. You can read labels—and you will have to do just that if you don't plan to cook everything from scratch. Dextrose, sucrose, and starch should immediately stand out like brilliant neon signs. Words such as *honey* and *syrup from corn* or *cane* should become the reddest of flags or flashing lights signaling danger. You can learn to work with the menu in any restaurant. Waitpeople *will* go to the kitchen to question chefs—however reluctantly they head in that direction. You *can* get vegetables or salad instead of rice and potatoes. You're paying the bill, and you can insist on getting what you want.

It doesn't take much to get started, and it takes just a little more strength to keep going one day at a time. You wouldn't have survived fibromyalgia, fatigue, and all your other symptoms if you were weak. You wouldn't have picked up this book and read this far if you didn't really want to get better. You have more courage than you think. All you need to do now is take the first step, and then the second, and then just keep going!

CHAPTER 6

❖

Diabetes

Diabetes is not just feeling dehydrated from your kidneys trying to eliminate excess sugar in the blood, it is also *pain.* I found this out recently. I thought I was experiencing a major FM relapse. I hurt *all over.* *Then* I tested my blood sugar. The genetic hammer has fallen. I am a diabetic. Controlling my blood sugar with a low-carbohydrate diet not only eliminates the intense exhaustion so common with diabetes, it also eliminated a lot of muscle pain I assumed was fibromyalgia. I thought hypoglycemia was bad. Diabetes is worse. Carbohydrate restriction is the answer to controlling both.

—*Kathleen S., Panama City, Florida*

If you've read the preceding chapters in order, you've been sequentially introduced to fibromyalgia and related conditions that can arise from the systemwide shortage of energy it causes.

We've tried to present them in a logical order, the way they might occur in patients. First we'd expect to see hypoglycemia, followed by excess weight and insulin resistance (with or without hyperglycemia); then might follow its cohort, full-blown diabetes. It's the nature of these interrelated abnormalities to follow one another in a not-altogether-orderly progression. If unchecked, all successfully diminish energy production, though diabetes is by far the most malicious. Unless it's carefully controlled, unlike fibromyalgia, it inevitably leads to permanent and irreversible damage. If treated, however, diabetes can be easily managed, as we've seen with many of our patients.

Over the years you've become well acquainted with the symptoms of fibromyalgia. Though they change and appear in different combinations, you've gotten to know them pretty well. We've reviewed the overlapping symptoms mimicked by hypoglycemia, and the regional aches or stiffness added by obesity. Now we will discuss diabetes and the complaints that come with it. Probably the best known of these is increased urination, which can certainly make a fibromyalgic's propensity for bladder infections worse. Blurred vision, fluid retention, and irritable bowel attacks are other early symptoms that obviously overlap those of fibromyalgia and even hypoglycemia. Given a bit of time, diabetes will affect the entire body. For this reason, the effects of hypoglycemia, obesity, and diabetes make it impossible to attribute a given symptom to any one of the coexisting illnesses. This trio certainly adds significant problems to the numerous ones caused by fibromyalgia. And when diabetes is present along with fibromyalgia, the depletion of energy is dramatically worse.

If you've got elevated blood sugars, you have long since

given in to your carbohydrate craving. This repeated yielding may already have seriously altered your once smooth body functions. It takes a lot of mismanagement to drag a healthy body into significant damage. You now have to contend with the bigger problem of diabetes. Unlike hypoglycemia, this one isn't ushered in with a bunch of scary symptoms. It takes its sweet time to do its sour work.

Once you understand what diabetes is and what causes it, you can begin to make diet and lifestyle changes that may help reverse the disease and help you reclaim your energy.

WHAT IS DIABETES?

I am a fifty-year-old six-foot, one-inch male who is active and owns his own business. I've never even broken a bone. I don't smoke, and I drink in moderation. Ten years ago when I turned forty I had a routine physical because I thought it was the responsible thing to do. My blood work revealed a blood sugar of 350. The doctor didn't seem to regard this as a major problem; he didn't even tell me I was diabetic. He said that I would have to change the way I eat because my blood sugar was high. He told me to see his dietician. She believed in moderate amounts of foods including carbohydrates and showed me lots of plates with plastic food on them to demonstrate what a proper portion was. I had no idea I was in any kind of serious trouble.

—*Lou M., Los Angeles, California*

Diabetes is divided into two broad groups. The first, Type I, is primarily a juvenile disease, though it occasionally comes on later in life. The other, as you'd suspect, is labeled Type II, the adult-onset variety. There are also variations in this classification that we'll ignore since they contribute nothing to this discussion. What follows is fairly basic. We suggest that those of you well versed in diabetes read swiftly through this section and pay more attention to the part titled What's the Solution?

Does the type really matter? You bet it does. Type I is a serious problem that isn't easily treated or controlled. Because it strikes young people, it evokes strong emotional reactions from both the parents and the patient. It's frightening because it arrives so suddenly and is foreboding in its implications. It's the type most feared because of its complications. Such patients will have to use insulin by injection, subscribe to meticulous, lifelong control, and prepare themselves for many medical misadventures.

Type I is relatively easy to diagnose. It hits hard and fast, and the patient becomes abruptly ill. It usually appears with a prostrating cluster of symptoms that may include nausea, vomiting, weakness, weight loss, heavy urination, flushing, and fever. The doctor realizes this is a very sick person and immediately orders blood tests. Results in, alarmed laboratory personnel phone urgently to announce their findings of extremely high plasma glucose. The patient is treated expeditiously and appropriately with insulin, usually with resounding and dramatic success. It's the story of diabetic ketoacidosis—a true medical emergency, possibly lethal if not speedily recognized. This type of diabetes is caused by the destruction of pancreatic tissue, and cannot be repaired by diet, exercise, or weight loss. These patients must always take insulin, though their insulin needs will be less and their blood sugars will be better controlled if they follow a careful diet and get regular exercise. Type I diabetics will always be diabetic; diet and exercise may tighten control of their illness, but they will not make it go away.

Type II is a more gentle disease, at least in its presentation. It develops slowly and rather insidiously, which allows more time for patient education and, hopefully, compliance. There are approximately fifteen million people already diagnosed with this type in the United States. Many others are wandering about who don't have a clue they have a problem. Not just by chance, this condition most often appears in tandem with obesity its most glaring harbinger. But given time, the vast majority of patients will unfortunately segue into several of the well-known complications of diabetes. The good news is that Type II *is* responsive to diet and exercise. Given the proper directions, these patients can avoid the ravages of the illness, if they only will comply.

Since the adult disease has a sneaky onset, it's often difficult to know exactly when it started in any given patient. The American Diabetes Association currently draws a line for the cutoff of normal *fasting* blood sugar. Eight hours without food or caloric drink is required, so samples are usually taken in the early morning. The magic number is 126 milligrams per deciliter. It's often expressed on laboratory reports as 126 mg./dl. They have further amended this with the statement that any blood sugar above 108 mg./dl. might be an indicator of diabetes. We consider ourselves fortunate indeed when we catch patients with such a scant elevation, because that signals an early stage of the disease. Usually we aren't that lucky; patients generally present with much higher levels. The reason for this is simple: If blood tests are ordered because patients have developed suspicious symptoms, their disease has usually progressed to some degree.

Whenever it's made, the diagnosis of adult-onset diabetes is an ill omen concerning what will eventually follow. Because the body struggles desperately to maintain metabolic balance, it exposes few clues initially. This means that by the time chemically detectable changes reveal themselves, some damage is already done. Even then, ominous subtleties only peak up like the tip of an iceberg. This explains our urgency in stressing the necessity for early detection. Current thinking is that it's never too soon to apply the label *diabetes* in lieu of some euphemism like "your sugar is a little high."

Endocrinologists know that the illness is already under way even at the earliest signs of tissue resistance to the hormone insulin. This is why we think it's wise to diagnose impending diabetes at the very inception of what's called insulin resistance. It's not particularly difficult to describe what these words mean. Insulin has direct effects on most organs and structures of the body. Like all hormones, it's formed in one location (certain cells in the pancreas) and travels to distant sites carrying specific instructions. Once it arrives at its destination, it instructs cells to perform some kind of chemical reaction. This response varies, depending upon which type of cell remains willing to accept programmed commands.

As time goes by, reluctant cells simply refuse to serve as obediently as in the past. With time, their defiance becomes overt and is confirmed when insulin rises abnormally high in the bloodstream. The situation is similar to handling a disobedient child. Even though your soft-spoken order was clearly audible, he or she stubbornly pretends not to hear. To counter this, you raise your voice to command immediate attention. The pancreas, the organ where insulin is manufactured, is a bit like that. When it first perceives rebellion in previously subservient tissues, it barks a little louder by extruding progressively more insulin. Initially this may work to elicit the desired response, and the blood sugar remains under control. Like children too frequently snapped to attention by repetitive shouting, however, cells eventually pretend not to hear even the loudest chemical commands. If this sounds like war, it is. We'll address this struggle again when we get to our next section.

Before we leave this topic, we'd like to spend a little longer on our definition. We know that physicians will quarrel with our simplistic designation of diabetes as synonymous with insulin resistance. In response, we'd answer that we think there's a problem with the older tradition of diagnosing diabetes only after symptoms surface. This really is a bit late in such a potentially deadly game. As we see time and time again, an early counterattack assures a greater chance for total victory against any illness. The time-worn criteria of very high blood sugar and its appearance in the urine are late indications of an already long-standing abnormality.

Insulin resistance can't be identified in your doctor's office. It's not usually measured because of the stringent conditions required to uncover this subtle abnormality. Insulin levels have to be checked in a hospital research setting where everything is tightly controlled. It can be done, but the cost isn't justified for the small amount of information it provides. After all, an abnormal fasting blood sugar is sufficient proof that cells are not responding to insulin as they should. The pancreas is like a biologic sensitive blood glucose monitor designed to read blood glucose levels. It normally pours precise amounts of insulin into the bloodstream in full harmony with changes in plasma glucose. Any failure to obey can be spotted in the simple fact that a patient's fasting blood value is too high. Higher-than-expected results show clearly that insulin has lost control. This means any reading above the accepted 126 mg./dl. is a sign that your body isn't able to get glucose out of your bloodstream as well as it should. Health professionals are gradually realizing this. If retesting confirms the abnormality, the diagnosis is diabetes. The American Diabetes Association now says it's so, and we heartily agree.

There's a major hurdle to widespread acceptance of such a simple definition of diabetes, and it has nothing to do with a patient's health. Once a person is diagnosed with diabetes, the self-serving insurance industry raises a red flag. It doesn't matter to insurance companies that you had only a slightly elevated sugar, which you quickly learned to control. It doesn't matter that you may still run marathons and work hard to keep your weight down. You'll be forever assessed higher health premiums unless you belong to a good-size group policy through your employer for the rest of your life. You can appreciate the concern this situation fosters in both patients and physicians. It's every doctor's goal to make an early diagnosis if damage is to be avoided. Yet this noble effort is counterproductive if insurance costs jump or the patient becomes uninsurable.

So what is the truth? When is it too soon to consider that an abnormal glucose equates to diabetes? In our mind, never. Unless there's a lab error, any rise is at the very least an omen. You can blame it on pregnancy, or stress, or temporary weight gain, but isn't it better for you to immediately accept your insulin resistance and do something about it? It's never too soon to begin taking care of yourself. At the elevated fasting blood sugar stage, physicians could actually avoid using the diagnostic word *diabetes* in patient charts. It wouldn't be much of a stretch to simply label the situation *carbohydrate intolerance*. Perhaps the term *diabetes* should be used only when medical intervention would normally be required. Launching one more barb, we hope someone wiser than an insurance bureaucrat knows when that moment arises. Avoiding further debate or semantics, let's proceed with what really counts for your health.

WHAT'S THE PROBLEM?

> Fatigue and I have finally come to an understanding. It's taken me years to realize when I feel tired and I've exhausted all the possibilities: not enough sleep, too much exertion, I know my blood sugar is too high. The first time this was brought home to me was when I was working on a job where, as the weeks went by, I was less and less inclined to go to work. I was despondent because I couldn't figure out why I had lost my enthusiasm for the job. I had given in to all the usual excuses: creative block, oncoming cold, I need a mental health day, et cetera. I went to the doctor and he did blood tests, and my blood sugar was high. I went on the diet and in only a few days I was feeling like my old self. I was scared I had lost my spark for living. Instead I had blown out that spark by eating too many carbohydrates and sugar.
>
> —*Lou M., Los Angeles, California*

There are approximately one million cell clusters in the pancreas that form well-demarcated islands. They were first described more than two hundred years ago by a German physician and are named for him, the islets of Langerhans. Powerful hormones are produced within those tiny atolls from an assortment of cells within those structures. One is called the beta cell, the source of the hormone insulin. Other types make their own messengers that either support or counter insulin effects.

As we've already discussed, Type I diabetes has a clear-cut cause. This so-called juvenile-onset type represents a wipeout of beta cells. The body suddenly mounts an all-out attack to destroy them. What induces this irresponsible destruction is sometimes uncertain. Usually it's when antibodies, the body's seek-and-destroy missiles, are created to fight off some virus. Insulin-producing cells are mistakenly perceived as enemies. Possibly it's because they resemble the enemy, but the beta cells are attacked and killed by the body's own forces, victims of friendly fire.

Once destroyed, such specialized tissues don't grow back. All kinds of tricks to correct this situation are currently being researched. So far, nothing's worked for very long. Transplants are costly and require potent drugs to suppress the body's immune system for life. Hope lies in impressive work in progress using fetal pancreatic cells. Even more promising are attempts to grow stem cells, basic little units that haven't yet decided on their career in the body. These cells could produce any structure the body makes. If they could be extracted and prodded by using proteins we call growth factors, new beta cells could be manufactured.

Type II diabetes, or diabetes mellitus, by contrast, allows a much greater opportunity for timely reversal in its initial stages. Whereas Type I demands considerable physician intervention, the adult disease can be totally managed by compliant patients. Though guidance is essential initially, physicians, their assistants, and diet professionals should later assume secondary roles. From then on, patient skills can completely avert most of the complications that are often perceived to be the normal progression of the disease.

There are deep impressions forever emblazoned in the minds of doctors who train or teach in diabetes clinics. Simply hearing the word conjures up vivid images for physicians. As dramatic as this might sound, it is, unfortunately, the truth. According to type, diabetics have particular weight characteristics. Type I is most often trim. Lean Type II diabetics do exist, but only as a glaring minority. Unfortunately, many of those slender ones end up using insulin, since they're often latent juvenile varieties. The dominant image of Type II is overweight. Ironically, the overweight Type II diabetic is the most salvageable. If you're one of these, no matter how you mourn your fate, you're one of the lucky diabetics. You've got the best chance for repair: You can completely erase every trace of your illness except the genetic propensity, which you can keep in abeyance if you're willing to change some things about your lifestyle.

Let's ignore the fact that most patients with early-phase Type II diabetes consistently skip very lightly over what their doctors try to tell them. If you have this type of diabetes and you choose to read on, you're certainly one of those for whom we are writing. We know that at first you feel no ill effects from your changing sugar metabolism. You may notice only the fact that you're not as energetic as you used to be, but you're probably tempted to ascribe this to the passing of years. Yet it's only a matter of time, if your disease is improperly managed, before you find more than simple energy losses ravaging your system.

The body is a survivor, and so are its component cells. Even when injured, they posture themselves defensively, thinking they can save themselves from permanent damage. They have all kinds of adaptive processes they display while waiting for recovery. It's in these stages that we can direct our most effective attempts at restoration. Dead cells can't be revived, so we must heal the sick ones if we are to save you from full-blown diabetes and an energy loss you can never repair.

Let's revisit insulin resistance, because understanding it is so crucial. In the initial stages of diabetes, insulin is still being exported from the pancreas, and it continues to find its way into the circulation. It eagerly locks in on the same cell wall receptors it has always visited in the past. To outside observers, at least, the beta cells appear to be doing the job for which they were designed. Why then do other cells rebel? Why this sudden reluctance to cooperate with insulin's message? As we've already touched upon, the problem begins in specific cells far removed from the pancreas.

Before the advent of resistance, fat cells were content and fully complied with insulin's instructions. They were always eager to accept every little fat package sent their way. This is the mechanism that allowed the body to survive when food was scarce. In some people, however, this old-fashioned obedience has gone on too long and to excess. Most of their fat cells have stuffed themselves with all of the delivered cargo, and have now become too large. Contoured by too many deliveries, the cells suddenly seem to realize they should have refused to accept them a long time ago. In danger of no longer being able to function properly, they understand it's time for new behavior, an entirely different biochemical posture.

We aren't in the habit of thinking of fat cells as endocrine glands. Yet now we know they have their own hormonal system to let the brain know things aren't going well. Better than this, many other tissues in the body eavesdrop on chemical conversations. If they validate the fat cells' complaints, they react favorably and speak out.

The brain isn't exactly impervious to this mounting defiance. It easily interprets the messages sent by the rebellious fat cells and hears the confirmation sent by their allies. The brain realizes that one of its staunchest allies, insulin, has become victimized by altogether too many dietary indiscretions. Remember, the brain is very protective of its glucose supply. Despite warnings of total warfare being delivered by the overloaded fat cells, the brain becomes an arrogant commander and refuses to listen. Bloodborne pleas from besieged fat cells are totally ignored. This is why we continue to feel the need to eat even when our body has overloaded fat cells. Hunger pangs and craving notices are sent to the taste buds as before; satiety is never reached. The brain hasn't learned that it lives in an age of plenty.

Adding to the problem, one recent medical paper has reported a disconcerting finding. Offspring of mothers who were diabetic during pregnancy carry a higher risk for developing both obesity and Type II diabetes. This hand-in-hand future threat is shared by the mother. The trend was not so for children born of diabetic fathers. It would seem that mother's genes and bad habits send hormonal curses to create lifelong hazards for her tiny embryo. Equally disturbing are reports that most members of diabetic families are insulin resistant. In short, insulin resistance in our era of plentiful food supply is an epidemic, and we all should be alert to its cause and progression. It is no secret, after all, that diabetes has reached epidemic proportions in the developed world, and is now rearing its ugly head in developing nations and growing children.

WHAT'S THE SOLUTION?

> I kept ignoring the hypoglycemia diet for as long as I could. Finally I decided I might have a problem with blood sugar, and also needed to lose weight, so I started the diet. After three months on the diet I was still feeling and having some low blood sugar episodes. Discussed it with my doctor, who had me do the glucose tolerance test. Guess what—I'm not hypoglycemic, I'm diabetic. I have continued on the diet now and my fasting blood sugar is always in the seventies and eighties and I've never had to take any type of medication. Just to have my blood sugar under control has made a huge difference in my life.
>
> —*Sharon C., Charlotte, North Carolina*

We're the ones who must mediate a cease-fire between our fat cells and our brains. We must somehow put an end to the rapid-sequence insulin waves. To succeed, we've got to get insulin to withdraw if we're going to resolve the conflict and emerge victorious and in control of our energy. The alternative is to join the current epidemic of adult-onset diabetes.

First of all, fat cells must be shrunken into a submissive size. They just can't do this without curbing insulin onslaughts. Not only will they comply once you start cooperating, but so will your muscles. Since these two tissues are the largest targets for insulin, their restored compliance alone can solve the problem. Skinnier fat and leaner muscle cells will agree to a renewed partnership if the armistice terms are reasonable.

We suspect you can already guess at how to accomplish this. Obviously, to stop your pancreas from releasing insulin, you'll have to reinvent your diet. As we've seen time and time again in these pages, carbohydrates are the main stimulants by causing the blood sugar to rise dramatically within minutes of ingestion. For this reason, carbohydrates are precisely what you'll have to give up. At this juncture, if you say, "I won't do it," and you mean it, skip to the next chapter. When the day comes and your symptoms take over your life, you can flip back to this record.

As we discussed in chapter 3, on hypoglycemia, the beta cells aren't aroused very much if you avoid sugars and starches. True, you have already damaged some of them by the time you have elevated blood sugar readings, but others of them are only stunned or injured. If you reform in time, these remaining cells might be able to handle a more restrictive diet naturally. This will save you a lot of hassles: daily blood sugar monitoring, constantly trying to establish the proper dosage of some risky medications, and, for a few lucky ones, those unpleasant injections of insulin.

Prior to 1921, diabetes was always fatal—the diagnosis was a death sentence. The symptoms had long been known, the name diabetes mellitus is from the Greek phrase meaning "to siphon sugar." As early as the 1600s, physicians knew the pancreas was involved and in subsequent years they had even figured out that lack of a hormone they named *inulin* (from the islets) and then *insulin,* was the cause. Before Banting and Best discovered a way to isolate insulin from the pancreas, people were kept alive longer using the only tool at hand, that is, diet.

However, "kept alive longer" usually meant only a matter of months. That's why their discovery was so monumental. It was one of the great findings in medical history and certainly equal to the discovery of penicillin. There are about fifteen million people alive today as a direct result—the availability of insulin has saved exponentially more lives than even the polio vaccine.

Once insulin became available throughout the world, which was as early as 1922, these life-saving injections were enthusiastically adopted and food restrictions were eased a bit. The tether was loosened on carbohydrate restraints, and diabetics were given more freedom in their diets. The strict black-and-white admonitions that *you-can-eat-this-and-none-of-that* were thrust aside, because daily survival no longer depended upon absolute perfection. Many food assortments were added in an attempt to ease what seemed only boring choices. The reasoning was simple: Let them have some sugar and starch, and we'll add a little more insulin to cover the indiscretions. Unfortunately, that was based on erroneous reasoning, and it greatly weakened what should have remained a firm interdiction.

During the early decades that followed the discovery of insulin, physicians simply winked at what was presumed to be only occasional cheating by patients. Despite this new laissez-faire attitude, simple sugars were kept off limits for most diabetics. Doctors began thinking this was sufficient to promote better ancillary health measures. They secretly hoped that patients would exercise dietary restraints *most* of the time. However, such relaxed measures seemed too liberal for some endocrinologists to willingly accept. Wiser words were frequently uttered by some leading centers dissenting from the newly sanctioned laxity. Not many diabetics and only a few physicians heeded these hard-liners. It was much more pleasant all around just to allow patients an easier dietary route.

This eat-anything-inject-more-insulin diet stopped controlling many Type II diabetics, but physicians were not immediately outmaneuvered. Various oral medications were developed that prod the already struggling pancreas to produce more insulin. Thus, some people can stave off insulin injections for a few years, but this approach is doomed to eventual failure when the pancreas can no longer respond. Newer compounds now being marketed closely mimic insulin activity if sufficient hormone remains available, that is, if the pancreas is not too damaged. These help by lowering the tissue resistance we've discussed. Unfortunately, stimulating already struggling cells of the pancreas works for only so long. Eventually it becomes like beating a dead horse. Huge numbers of adult-onset diabetics will still end up requiring insulin if longevity proves their good fortune.

Unless they adhere to dietary restrictions—insulin or oral medications notwithstanding, most Type II diabetics continue their alarming weight gain. Insulin, the storage hormone, forces on the pounds even while bringing sugar levels down. Thus, the disease eventually becomes literally too big to handle. Blood sugar inexorably rises to further impose what is known as glucose toxicity. More insulin-producing cells are destroyed from this type of poisoning. The islets of Langerhans glaze over with a gel-like substance called amyloid. On the pancreas, these deposits stand out like so many stones marking the graves of defunct beta cells.

Finally it's too late to succeed with simple dieting. Outside help from medical personnel now becomes more structured and invasive. Death is avoided by using insulin injections two or three times a day. At this point, a very stringent protocol is mandatory. Oddly enough, diabetics must now listen to the same dietary counseling—the exact words—previously ignored. With the addition of insulin, timing its use to the type of food is crucial. Meals must be eaten at regular intervals, and even snacks consumed at well-defined moments. Calories are precisely allocated in tailored ratios different for breakfast, lunch, and dinner. The proper amount of insulin must be calculated exactly and administered at the correct time or symptoms from hypoglycemia can occur with a vengeance. Patients who previously refused self-control now find it thrust upon them. Many now comply only because of their doctor's dire warnings and sheer physical discomfort.

Years of accumulated data have clearly shown the life-extending virtues of tightly controlling diabetes. Insulin must be adjusted according to food intake, using a little device to self-test blood glucose. Three or four times per day, fingers are lanced to ooze the requisite drop of blood needed for that determination. A log of the results is kept for physicians to study. In this way, insulin can be adjusted to accommodate dietary compliance and activities. Recommendations are aimed at confining blood sugar within predetermined ranges. Patients were once counseled to inject insulin twice daily. But we know that blood sugar is better controlled with a precise amount of several kinds of insulin taken on a schedule that mimics hormone release. Well-based, scientific data suggest that it's best to mete out no more insulin than necessary. For ideal results, patients must meticulously adhere to this slightly time-consuming and exacting protocol.

Unfortunately, even this late in the story the recommended tight discipline is not readily acceptable for most Type II diabetics. This is not too surprising, since these are usually the same individuals who steadfastly rejected previous dietary advice. What? Give up pastas and potatoes? To them, the promise of better health and energy down the road doesn't seem worth the sacrifice. And it never might.

Our story is incomplete. Can the diabetic, insulin syringe in hand, now live happily ever after? Unfortunately, this is not usually the case, even when a patient tries his best, since our methods of introducing the hormone and techniques for exact dosing remain primitive. We lack the technology, and often the patient's cooperation, for providing perfect and scrupulous control. Since the pancreas normally releases insulin directly into certain abdominal veins, the initial diversion is to the liver. In contrast, the subcutaneous method of injection that we have to use for self-administered insulin injections ignores normal physiology. Large amounts are suddenly introduced and make their way into parts of the circulation that aren't the body's preferred system of dispersal. This method by necessity ignores the inborn wisdom of the liver and its delicate tissue monitoring. Even with our most advanced modern contraptions and fancy new kinds of insulin, much is lacking, and there's no substitute for our own natural pancreas.

Thus, even with good behavior and conscientious management there is accelerated damage in diabetes. Glucose floats in the blood as tiny energy-supply packets, and working tissues are normally avid for sugar. But when insulin is in short supply, cellular entry is denied and sugar remains adrift.

Sugars are sticky, as you know from touching a candy bar. It's a bit similar in the bloodstream, where glucose is attracted to proteins that compose various structures. The walls of some cells become either leaky where they should be tight or sealed when they should be porous. Enzymes and hormones also get tagged in the process and suffer minuscule alterations in function. Their normally swift and precise actions become slightly gooey.

There are a lot of other little saboteurs lurking about in our bodies. They're quite varied in their appearances and often disguised, rendering them difficult to recognize. We identify them as reactive oxygen species, and unfortunately they are intent on reaping destruction wherever they're produced. Oxygen has to be chemically welded to some types of receptive molecules to avoid cellular damage. A lack of insulin unleashes some of the restraints and weakens the body's protective defenses. That's why antioxidants are often recommended in the form of vitamin B_6, folic acid, and vitamin E for each of us, not only diabetics.

A little earlier in this book we touched on the metabolic syndrome, known as Syndrome X, in the pages on obesity. It's time to mention it again, because all the symptoms appear to be associated with high insulin levels. These include abdominal fat deposits, high blood pressure, and a disturbance in blood fat levels, or lipids. High cholesterol, high triglycerides, and low HDL (good cholesterol) levels appear on blood test results. It is this combination that seems to dramatically increase the risk of cardiovascular disease. Since they're all so closely linked to insulin resistance, you should know that to control your insulin problem is to vanquish the others as well.

We wouldn't be cruel enough to depict such menacing outcomes were there no alternatives. If you're already an early and overweight diabetic, you're welcome to join those for whom we are writing. There are many books on how to manage diabetes once you have it. We have less interest in coping because we know you can avoid a head-on collision if you'll listen now.

If you're obese and insulin resistant or diabetic, glucose testing should have taught you one important thing: Ingesting sugars or complex starches raises blood sugar. The same low-carbohydrate diet we advocated in the previous two chapters provides the saving grace again in this one. Stop eating carbohydrates and you'll simply require less insulin. Deprived of carbohydrates, the body will have to turn to fat for energy. It will not only use up everything you eat, but also coax progressively more fat out of its storage place inside fat cells to make energy. Though the chemistry is not quite that simplistic, you will lose weight and inches. Your pancreas will be given time to relax and restore whatever function remains. If you start early enough, you'll escape lifelong dependence on medication and daily blood sugar testing.

That's how one diet fits snugly into our well-designed metabolic health. Restricting carbohydrates, you can lose weight as well as correct hypoglycemia, insulin resistance, and the hyperglycemia of diabetes. And as a fibromyalgic, you will have more energy. Can you trust this? You bet you can! Go ahead, be skeptical, it's healthy. Try the experiment: Work with your doctor *and* do what these pages say. See what happens.

For losing weight, use the diet outlined in chapter 5, on obesity. Once you've lost what you want, use the diet in chapter 3, on hypoglycemia, because the purpose of the HG diet is to control blood sugar. Be prepared for a verbal assault from family, friends, and possibly physicians. Each of them will probably raise the same issue. What will happen to your cholesterol and other fats? The answer to this question is in chapter 8, about lipids.

You've read how to correct fibromyalgia by reversing your symptoms and can find more detailed information in our book *What Your Doctor May Not Tell You About Fibromyalgia*. You've learned how to control hypoglycemia and resultant hormonal releases that result in fatigue. We've given you early warnings of insulin resistance and the threat it poses. You know how all these conditions drain your energy and weigh down your body. Don't dismiss out of hand the beneficial effects weight loss would add. Even if you're already thin and diabetic, our diet will help you control your blood sugar levels. You already know the toll that high blood sugar levels take on your energy. It may even be possible to salvage some of your beta cells for use later down the line. If you can do this, you'll need less medication, and less intervention.

If you've read this far, you've come a long way. But there's still more. Further repairs may still be needed to reclaim and discover the benefits of having abundant energy. Look ahead. And keep reading.

CHAPTER 7

The Hormone Hoax

In their desperation to help, physicians and various medical practitioners have taken to inserting various amounts of hormones into the already mixed-up metabolism of the fibromyalgic patient. We've witnessed an entire spectrum: everything from the use of a single hormone in small or large amounts, to the use of combinations of two hormones in varied amounts, to a bunch of tiny assortments. We think it is important for you, the patient, to understand why this approach may in the long run actually *reduce* your energy.

From what we've seen daily in our practice, we think it's sadly become necessary to write these pages to warn the usually unsuspecting public. It is they who will too late discover the long-range ravages of these powerful chemicals when used as supplements. We know our words will often fall on deaf ears, because too many people believe that feeling better momentarily is synonymous with safety or "worth the risk." But is it? Read on, and make up your own mind, please.

In-your-face advertisements abound trying to sell hormone

supplements that promise victory against aging, enormous boosts to waning strength, and relief from precipitous fatigue. There's no question that various levels can be at the low or high range of normal in fibromyalgics. A battery of tests done by a well-meaning physician looking desperately for any abnormality to treat will often turn up one or two of these. Patient and doctor often seize upon these as something to "fix." But can you fix fibromyalgia by adding hormones to a system that can't make enough energy, and what happens when you do?

WHAT IS A HORMONE?

The word *hormone* is of Greek derivation, from the verb that means "to excite." A medical dictionary definition goes something like this: "An internal secretion produced in and by one of the endocrine glands that is carried by the bloodstream or body fluids to other parts of the body where it has a specific physiological effect." More simply put, hormones are biochemical products of various glands that are transported to instigate action in a different area of the body. They're messengers!

Hormones carry very significant and specific instructions that have awesome effects. They command immediate respect even though they often allow for actions to be delayed. Once even a small amount enters a system, there's a cascading effect. Unlike some of the other systems we've discussed, this isn't warfare. Quite the contrary; it's total cooperation in the best of biologic sequences. It's skillful diplomacy at its most graceful.

How many hormones are there? Where do their receptors lie? These are mostly unanswerable questions at this stage of technology, which is part of the dilemma when we use them. This is what we work with every day in our practice as endocrinologists.

The total number of hormones accrues faster than we ever imagined—new ones are discovered almost annually. This is truly an exciting field because it keeps asking, "Why?"

Hormones Carry Messages, But Each Is Different

Every hormone has a different shape and chemical structure. We bunch them into certain classifications depending on some dominant features. One category whose name you'll recognize immediately is the group known as steroids. That's a family name for members with names you'll also immediately recognize. Among those are estrogen, progesterone, testosterone, cortisone, and DHEA. Some synthetic steroids have an evil connotation earned because of abuses by athletes. Others have bad reputations because they're believed to have a profound effect on behavior: testosterone and estrogen, for example. A less well-known group is known as peptides or polypeptides. They're assembled in distinctive patterns so that each particular biochemical linkage will be instantly recognized by a highly personal and exclusive receptor that lies in wait. This is because hormones work through receptors, as a diplomat might work through a translator. Without receptors to carry their message into the cell, a hormone cannot work. This is why hormones can only work on certain cells; without the medium there is no message.

We don't intend to discuss all the well-known hormones, because not all of them have relevance in this treatise on fatigue. We'll particularly avoid the newer family members, because too little is known about them. In any case, many have not yet been synthesized so they're unavailable as supplements, making them safe from inappropriate use for the moment. Others are well enough known but don't serve endangered functions in the body.

They're safely tucked into various tissues and haven't yet been bottled for injection or swallowing. The few we've chosen to discuss are those most frequently prescribed and subject to abuse by both patients and physicians. Mishandled, they further deplete the energy and stamina of struggling fibromyalgics, and that is the problem we're going to address.

Why Do We Need Hormones?

Hormones are produced and designed in mysterious patterns by the endocrine glands. Once their code is broken by researchers, they can be synthesized, or copied in laboratories, and it becomes tempting to use them. Since they are perfect copies of the natural messenger, suddenly it's possible for us to invade the inner recesses of a cell. It's as though the combination to a previously locked vault is made suddenly available. Having broken the secret code, we can send orders of our own.

It's the very prowess of hormones that makes them attractive. Both patients and physicians frequently fail to think that such potency might serve as a double-edged sword that should be wielded responsibly. Just having massive weapons in our arsenal is not an excuse to use them at every small provocation. We should remember that biologic dynamics are never simple, and every interjection has the potential for complications. Similar to a law of physics, every action demands a counterreaction. The effect of either ingesting or injecting a hormone is promptly reflected internally by some countermeasure. The other glands in the system don't stand idly by when the status quo is upset. You mess with one and not too surprisingly, the others often rise to protect. We'll face this repeatedly, and it is a problem that too few stop to consider.

THE THYROID—WHAT DOES THIS GLAND HAVE TO DO WITH ENERGY?

No other hormones are as widely prescribed—and for such dubious reasons—as the thyroid's. Because complaints of fatigue and weight gain are ubiquitous, patients and practitioners zero in on this gland. It's as though an underactive thyroid were the only possible culprit responsible for those ills.

The thyroid is a small, angel-wing- or shield-shaped gland. It's the body's metabolic thermostat that controls temperature and energy use. Like all endocrine glands, its power lies in its exports. Thyroid hormones have effects on all body processes and even on the rate at which organs should function. The human thyroid produces a number of hormones, but we're going to focus on two of them because so far they're the only ones that are abused.

The leading output of the thyroid is a hormone composed 95 percent of the amino acid tyrosine with four attached iodine molecules. This structure is reflected in its medical name, T_4. The remaining 5 percent is the same amino acid, this time carrying three iodine passengers. It's therefore referred to as T_3. Let's remember this important ratio of 95 to 5—nature's intended ratio for *human* thyroids.

When the thyroid gland is underproductive, we refer to the condition as hypothyroidism. Since the thyroid controls the metabolism of the body, an underactive thyroid means that the body becomes sluggish: Low energy and weight gain are the primary symptoms. Thus it's easy to see why many doctors and fibromyalgics think an underactive thyroid might be to blame for at least some of their symptoms.

Luckily, thanks to a superbly accurate test it's easy to check if you're hypothyroid. Blood is sampled to measure the level of thyroid stimulating hormone (TSH). As the name implies, this controller is not actually released by the thyroid, but is a messenger sent from the pituitary gland, the so-called master gland of the body. Though the thyroid is able to produce some hormone on its own, the majority of its output is dictated by the intensity of bombardment from the pituitary. If the thyroid gland becomes sluggish, more TSH sallies forth from the pituitary. Blood tests reflect this situation, showing an elevated level of TSH. In the reverse situation, if thyroid excesses enter the bloodstream the pituitary promptly compensates by releasing less TSH, so that the thyroid will curb its output. High TSH signifies thyroid underactivity; low TSH, overactivity or hyperthyroidism.

We should mention that there is a rare situation when the pituitary itself is sick. In this case, it does not adequately release one or more of its many hormones, including the TSH. Obviously, TSH will slowly or abruptly drop in the blood, and for a while the thyroid may maintain sufficient activity by itself, but this is a stopgap measure and won't work for long. Eventually, the so-called free T_4 will drop to an abnormally low level. When both the TSH and the thyroid hormones are low, physicians should be alert to this possibility. This condition is so rare that an endocrinologist should be consulted because further pituitary testing is vitally necessary. At this point, let's share one axiom repeatedly taught in medical schools: "If you rarely make a rare diagnosis, you will rarely miss a diagnosis!"

So What's the Problem?

Myths are being perpetuated on how best to treat a sick, underproductive gland. Patients are sometimes placed on thyroid hormones derived from cows and pigs known as thyroid extract, or Armour thyroid. These compounds are held in high esteem by those who prescribe them, and unsuspecting patients are told that these are "natural"—a term frequently used to inspire confidence that in reality means very little. In this case, especially, it is a most dubious claim unless you happen to be a pig or a cow who has an underactive thyroid gland.

A few paragraphs back we described the mix of T_4 and T_3 produced by human thyroid glands. It should go without saying that what's normal for cows and pigs may not be what's normal for us humans. Animals make a different mix of the two hormones—approximately 15 to 25 percent T_3. You'll recall that humans, in contrast, produce about 5 percent T_3. Ask yourself, then, why we should represent animal products as natural replacements for human hypothyroidism. The amazing part of this is that the precise human hormones have been expertly synthesized and are readily available in many, many different potencies. Levo-thyroxine (T_4) and tri-iodothyronine (T_3) are the true *natural* hormones, the ones the human thyroid generates.

In humans, we don't normally supplement T_3 because it isn't necessary. The reason is that our liver and some other tissues normally convert T_4 to T_3 as needed. For this reason, it's customary to replace deficient thyroid output with only T_4 and allow the system to make its own necessary conversions. Some debate has opened up on the need for adding a small amount of T_3 to supplement T_4 replacement therapy. The problem with this idea is that it's impossible to discern how much to give. When thyroid hormones are extraneously administered, blood measurements only reflect how much T_4 or T_3 is running loose in the bloodstream. We have no sure way of knowing what all of the various tissues might have scooped up for their own use. Only our own internal monitors, the pituitary and the adjacent brain hypothalamus, have the ability to make a precise interpretation of the rapid and minuscule variations on the bloodborne hormonal combinations. It's totally safe to say that if metabolism is meeting all the body's challenges, a normal blood TSH is the signal that these control tissues are content, and no outside interference is necessary. If some patients don't feel totally corrected using only T_4, a small amount of T_3 may certainly be added. The body will adjust production accordingly, and no harm will be done as long as the TSH remains in normal range.

The delicate nuances of very ordinary or rare thyroid diseases require the guidance of a physician who understands the interplay of the brain-pituitary-thyroid axis. He or she must take command and not allow patients to dictate treatment or determine dosages by how they *feel*. Once the TSH is sufficiently normal, whatever the initial disturbance, the thyroid problem is under control. The remaining complaints from the patient are not due to excess or insufficient thyroid hormone, and no further messing around should be contemplated or condoned beyond what we've been telling you. Read our previous chapters and learn for yourself how other illnesses cause identical complaints.

We are not suggesting that you should ignore an underactive thyroid. To do so permits an inexorable progression into hardening of the arteries, known as arteriosclerosis. Though cardiac effects are the prime concern, permanent damage may develop in other vital structures as circulation wavers. Even one year of hypothyroidism is conducive to some undesirable and permanent arterial changes. Cholesterol usually rises in hypothyroidism, furthering the assault on blood vessels. Beyond that, all tissues rely deeply on thyroid hormones for multiple, metabolic instructions.

Their needs should never be ignored. For this reason, it is essential that fatigue and other complaints that sound like hypothyroid be evaluated by a TSH blood test.

But there is a flip side to this equation, which reminds us that a perfect balance is desirable and, in fact, necessary. Excessive ingestion of thyroid hormones is extremely dangerous as well. Thyroid hormones are naturally designed to speed up most cellular processes. The entire body gets sparked into biochemical hyperactivity, because all systems share in this exhausting metabolic acceleration. Energy is furiously burned, much to the detriment of participating tissues. Such perpetual goading most immediately threatens the heart. Continuous overworking of this organ seriously impacts older patients, who may develop congestive heart failure because of their aging coronary arteries. Even more dangerous are altered cardiac rhythms that, sufficiently perturbed, act like irregular eggbeaters whipping blood inside heart chambers. Clots may form and be released, resulting in strokes when they lose their precarious hold on the heart wall. Even bones are impacted and instructed to relinquish some of their precious calcium stores, causing osteoporosis. This is too high a price to pay for a little additional energy or a slightly raised body temperature that, in any case, will not last.

Don't be duped by statements such as, "You have a normal level of _____ [any of the hormones], but it's a *low* normal." Normal is normal, so don't fall prey to pumping additional, unnecessary amounts into your metabolic equations. If you're lucky, and you know enough to keep your TSH in normal range, this exercise will only be a waste of your money. Let's give you an example. If a normal thyroid puts out 100 mcg. of T_4 per day, depend on the pituitary to monitor that production. If you now add one thyroid tablet that contains 50 mcg., the pituitary reads this new increment in the bloodstream. The master gland responsibly decreases TSH output. The thyroid dutifully responds by cutting T_4 releases in half, down by exactly 50 mcg. Add it up: You ingested 50 mcg. and got 50 mcg. less from the gland. The total, daily retrieval is the same 100 mcg. You've achieved nothing except forcing your own gland into semiretirement.

Do you have to second-guess your physician? We rarely advocate such action, but in the instance of thyroid and other hormone prescription practices, we're sorry that we must. As one of us completes fifty years in medicine, it's appallingly true that these days, hormones, particularly thyroid, are given almost promiscuously.

THE ADRENAL GLAND—WHAT IS IT AND HOW DOES IT IMPACT ENERGY PRODUCTION?

Each of us has two adrenal glands. They're situated atop each kidney, totally encased in a mound of fat, because nature takes great precautions with these vital structures. Thus situated, they're extremely well protected from damage by the adjacent ribs. Their strange shape—somewhat like a Napoleonic hat or bishop's miter—allows them to better fit the rounded top of the kidney. Each is only an inch or two long, and weighs a fraction of an ounce.

The adrenals have a rich blood supply, as befits their impressive functions within the endocrine system. Each gland is made up of two parts: the outer adrenal cortex and the inner medulla. The inner portion secretes the hormone adrenaline, which we've already discussed in chapter 3, on hypoglycemia. The adrenals also release a number of other hormones (more than forty) that we can mostly ignore for the purposes of this discussion. Many medications used for autoimmune or inflammatory diseases are synthetic models of adrenal steroids. In this section, we'll limit ourselves to hormones produced in the outer cortex, the so-called corticosteroids that so profoundly affect our metabolism and energy production.

These glands are important in their own right, but like the thyroid are largely subservient to commands emanating from the pituitary—and also, in this case, the hypothalamus. This section of the brain sends sequential instructions that result in perfectly timed releases of the adrenocorticotropic hormone, or ACTH. It enters the bloodstream and is cordially recruited by private receptors on adrenal cell surfaces.

Often the incoming news delivered by ACTH is a report about some kind of disturbing stress. Stimulated by this visitor, the adrenal cortex spews out a hormone of its own. It's a member of the large family we've briefed you about, the steroid clan. Though you'll recognize it best by the name *cortisone,* it's known in medicine as *cortisol,* or *hydrocortisone.*

Cortisol is an extremely potent and wide-ranging hormone, and has an effect on how our body uses incoming fuels: carbohydrates, fats, and proteins. Bingo! Here we are back in the realm of energy production! In times of duress, the body can release twenty times its basal amount of this hormone. It's promptly released when the body faces infection, trauma, surgery, emotional surges, and even exposure to excessive heat or cold. Since receptors friendly to cortisol are invested in the walls of most bodily structures, we know the extent of its domain.

Spurts of cortisol block the effects of insulin and cause the blood sugar to rise. The idea behind this process is to give you more energy, and it's this action of this hormone that is responsible for the dawn effect wherein our blood sugar rises to help us wake up and face the day. Cortisol also induces bone surfaces to break down to release calcium into the bloodstream. It steals amino acids from muscle storehouses and promotes their conversion to glucose in the liver. It coaxes fat cells into releasing their contents from reserve depots in the extremities, skin, and buttocks. Under its auspices, some fatty acids are plucked out for energy needs. These are all controlled responses designed to steal fuel from less essential functions and to meet a need that the body has perceived as an emergency.

Cortisol also impacts the immune system. It depresses the number and activity of immune cells. Under its command, various white cells partially disappear from the bloodstream. Since these are crucial to mounting an attack against infection, bacteria, viruses, and fungi meet far less resistance when they invade if cortisol levels are high. Antibody production also lags, because the liver continues its avid use of protein for conversion to glucose. As a result of this, rampant infections are an eminent danger of the prolonged use of cortisonelike hormones.

As if this were not enough, there are additional dangers with long-term use of steroids. Cataract formation accelerates, and blood pressure rises often to dangerous levels. Skin fragility can result in large wounds from relatively minor abrasive injuries when healing is compromised. Internal tissues are also affected, rendering patients poor surgical risks because of inadequate healing potential. Emotions become labile and swing rapidly ranging from depression to paranoia and from excitability to somnolence. There's a gradual progression to spreading arteriosclerosis and all the added morbidity that this entails. Osteoporosis is guaranteed, both from the theft of the bones' calcium and from an increased urinary excretion. Total body fatigue and weakness are rampant, where energy was initially increased. There's more, but this is enough to make our point.

Like Other Hormones, Cortisol Is Powerful

It's apparent by now that we hold the same healthy respect for cortisol (or cortisone) as we do for thyroid hormone. In the short term, they're safe and provide wonderful, therapeutic rewards. It's when considering long-term use that doctors must be extremely respectful. It's the duty of physicians to weigh any anticipated benefit against the distinct damage that longer therapy will eventually impose. We're in no way suggesting that cortisone-like drugs should be avoided at all cost. We're simply stressing that there must be a judicious evaluation of the anticipated price to be paid against the anticipated benefit. This is certainly a quid pro quo, but the bottom line is it's your life and you're both the payer and the payee.

Obviously we're not talking about avoiding these hormones altogether. We rail only against a stab-in-the-dark type of usage, not against using them when they're desperately needed. "I don't know what's wrong but let's try it" medical management is wrong when potent hormones are involved. An unfortunate example of this has surfaced in recent years with the profligate misdiagnosis of "adrenal insufficiency." From the darkness of ignorance and misdirection of inadequate testing, energy-depriving conditions are being attributed to the wrong villain. The rationale seems to be that a little bit of synthetic cortisone shouldn't hurt. Oh, but we believe it does!

Cortisol is particularly dangerous when given for too long

and at the wrong time of day, because it has what we call a diurnal variation. It begins to rise in the body and blood in the early hours before awakening—as we've seen—causing the blood sugar to rise and give us energy to wake up. That's why blood levels are highest in the morning upon arising, dip somewhat before lunch, rise slightly after eating, and drop off again by 4 P.M. For this reason, to least interfere with normal metabolism, cortisone-like drugs should be properly timed. Physicians who prescribe cortisone-like drugs should remember nature's ways. To do otherwise is to compound the damage of long-range use.

There's normally perfect harmony in the endocrine system. Pituitary control is very precise. If only a small amount of cortisone-like drug is ingested, the adrenals may not be totally shut down. However, larger or excessive amounts put the glands into deep sleep and will completely stop all internal production. Obviously, nothing will have been achieved as long as the medication exactly equals what the glands normally put out. Too much will put the glands in such depression that they won't recover for several months after the outside interference is stopped. The longer cortisol is taken, the longer the recovery time for your own glands. In the meantime, as your own glands slowly recover, your energy and stamina will be seriously compromised.

THERE'S ANOTHER ADRENAL HORMONE TO LOOK AT—DHEA

We promised you a discussion on two of the adrenal hormones, and here's the second. Another steroid is touted as the fountain of youth du jour. It is best known by its initials,

DHEA—dehydroepiandrosterone. Reach into the middle of that long chemical name and extract the letters *andro*. That root derivation refers to something masculine and is part of this hormone's long name for a good reason.

DHEA and its sulfate companion, DHEAS, are found in the bloodstream in greater amounts than any other hormone. When such levels circulate, it's usually a sign of the relative impotency of the hormone. Otherwise there wouldn't be a need for so much. Accordingly, it's considered a *pro*-hormone, suggesting that it needs to be worked on somewhere in the body to produce a more potent compound. Even after many years of study, the hormone hasn't yet been tied to any hugely important function. The skin and hair follicles convert it into male hormones, predominantly testosterone. The liver and other systems also have receptors for DHEA; conceivably, some other benefits may eventually be discovered. We do know that blood levels drop with aging along with those of the other sex hormones, estrogen, testosterone, and progesterone. By age eighty, most people display less than a fifth of the DHEA that existed during their peak production years of the twenties.

As a precursor of estrogen and testosterone, pumping extra DHEA into an aging body may be fraught with danger. Would it augment the already known increased risk of breast or prostate cancer? Besides that, as its name implies, it has effects that tilt more toward the male than the female side. Some women have already shown adverse consequences such as excessive, darkened hair growth on the face, breasts, and chest in a male pattern. Stopping the compound doesn't totally reverse this unwanted growth. Other outward signs of masculine effects, oily skin and acne, are sometimes accompanied by changes in blood lipids. More masculine patterns may appear such as a lower HDL and higher cholesterol. That's not good for women, who enjoy a lower risk of arteriosclerosis than do men, in part because of their better lipid distributions. How much DHEA will be converted to estrogen or to testosterone seems at the whim of the liver. No conversion ratios of either can be predicted as far as we yet know. Those who ingest it on a long-term basis should do so recognizing its uncertain peril at the current level of knowledge.

DHEA is a hormone in search of a destiny. There is no conclusive evidence that it rebuilds energy or retrieves lost youth. For patients whose adrenal glands have been destroyed or removed, cortisol is routinely provided for replacement therapy carefully used to imitate the secretion of the diseased gland. After such surgery, however, no attention has been given to restoring DHEA, and no ill effects have been apparent from this omission. It's safe to say, then, that the loss of this hormone has had no impact—no significant consequences have been witnessed. Is it a required hormone? Only time will tell. For now, current wisdom is not to risk a foray into the unknown, especially given negative studies that have just been published about sex hormone replacement.

HUMAN GROWTH HORMONE (HGH)

We have mentioned the mighty pituitary several times in this chapter. It's usually defined as the master gland that controls other endocrine tissues scattered all over the body. It's not entirely self-sufficient, because it takes orders from the brain.

Every pituitary hormone is a masterpiece of chemical ingenuity. Most are not yet commercially produced and are therefore not available for abuse. Unfortunately, this is no longer the case for the recently marketed human growth hormone (also known as HGH). It has widespread systemic consequences and a meticulous interplay with several other hormones. Though its benefits and drawbacks are fairly well known, inappropriate use is already not uncommon.

Growth hormone has an obvious function from birth until full maturity. Almost all our bodily structures have receptors that are built to receive and enact its commands. It continues to display its growth-promoting skills throughout our lives. It has subtle actions in adults that are mostly involved in tissue remodeling and repair. Many metabolic functions would greatly slow if we were suddenly deprived of its timely instructions—thus the temptation to speed them up by supplementing this hormone when it may not be needed.

Growth hormone must be prescribed by a doctor. It's usually given three or more times per week and *only by injection*. It cannot be taken orally, and any product that states otherwise is a scam. A major drawback is the cost of about two thousand dollars per month. Despite this, it is already being touted as a solution to aging, and there are wealthy or well-insured people who are using it for this purpose. Support for this stance is meager at best in males, unavailable for females, and awaits more facts before benefits can be confirmed.

Growth Hormone's Serious Side Effects

The following is not intended as a scare tactic. These words are warnings to enforce the notion that growth hormone should be used only for proper indications. Overproduction of this hormone from a pituitary tumor is the cause of a condition called acromegaly. All parts of the body enlarge under its steady onslaught. Unrestricted secretion thickens facial features as well as the hands, feet, and internal organs. Additionally, hypertension develops, diabetes ultimately appears, and the heart later succumbs as part of a generalized arteriosclerosis. If untreated, the fate of such patients is death by heart attack, stroke, or cancer that often arises from the colon.

For these reasons, growth hormone should not be added if pituitary production is normal. Continuous and inappropriate use eventually does its dirty work. Primarily because of antagonizing effects on insulin, full-blown diabetes may appear, slowly followed by the many documented ravages of that disease. Totally counterproductive as time passes, energy doesn't improve but actually wanes as these additional diseases are introduced.

Typical scams are already advertised using *oral* concoctions extracted from animals. Little matter that whatever growth hormone might remain in the preparation will be treated like any other protein food: It will be digested and totally broken into individual amino acids before absorption. At present, there is no effective oral preparation of growth hormone or growth hormone simulators. We might as well mention, while we're on this topic, the other various organ extracts, secretions, and enzymes. These all suffer the same fate as any other meat in their trip through the digestive system. We've avoided them in these pages since they are not hormones. However, an aside is justified because of their intrusion into our lives. Erroneously touted for almost any existing condition, they soak up all too many health dollars better saved for other medical needs. All are proteins, and only those designed for intestinal action will fulfill some mission before facing destruction.

THE BOTTOM LINE: HORMONES ARE POWERFUL AND NOT SIMPLE SOLUTIONS

Manufacturing drug companies strive to make patients and physicians feel there's a need for their products. Physicians desperately trying to help demanding patients will prescribe these compounds. In the end, it's your body, and you have to think the hardest about what you may be doing to it.

Demand diagnostic security when you're being urged to take potent medications. Hormones are necessities of life and, judiciously prescribed because of organ failure, are wondrous indeed. If your depleted energy comes from lack of some crucial compound, by all means replace it. Remember that your body seeks chemical balance. Adding wrong things for you, or some that you don't need, threatens that equilibrium and can rob you of the very improvement you were seeking. Don't let badly aimed hormonal darts further burst your partially deflated energy balloon.

❖

CHAPTER 8

Those Dirty Little Fats— Lipid Abnormalities

On television there's a commercial with a nice-looking older man diving into a swimming pool. He looks great, and women are looking at him appreciatively. Then type appears on the screen giving the man's height, weight, and finally his cholesterol level. It's astoundingly high, and the point is that he looks great and you'd never know something is wrong with him. That's the problem—it's just like fibromyalgia! You don't look sick, but inside you are.

—*Steve S., Los Angeles, California*

As we launch into the effects of fats on our systems, please remain focused on our dedication to energizing fibromyalgia. We've already alluded to the impact of genes on our metabolic processes. Just as genetic frailties assert themselves in fibromyalgia, they're also heavily involved in fat disposal. If you're predisposed to these lipid problems, you will struggle with your metabolism in much the way a hypoglycemic will battle with carbohydrates. Far too many people inherit errant mechanisms for absorption of nutrients or at least those that malfunction when our food supply is too plentiful. Food may be the source for all energy production, but the vast majority of us can't load everything we'd like into our diets. We really already know we can't eat our way throughout life without adverse consequences. Now come the equally monstrous errors in fat disposition and the damaging influence of their by-products. Like the other chapters in this book, this one also has relevance to restoring energy.

We've visited some other genetic pitfalls when we delved into hypoglycemia, obesity, and diabetes. Each of these issues is inexorably connected to the types of food we eat, and each has an obvious and immediate effect on our energy levels. This chapter is a little different because it's about fat metabolism. Lipid abnormalities cause no ripples in our energy waves until later in life. Yet they do eventually damage and take an insidiously heavy toll. We'll point our fingers in turn at the easily measured cholesterol, triglycerides, HDL, and calculated LDL. You've already met some of these interesting fellows and probably recognize their names. Our discussion may be of some interest even to those endowed with normal numbers. Though we hope you'll read along, this chapter is directed primarily at the less fortunate among us.

We've tossed the above lipid labels at you, but do you actually know what they mean? If you're over forty, your doctor has probably checked them a few times and read you the results. You have a good idea what cholesterol is all about. You may even know the exact value found on your last test.

If it happened to be higher than normal, was it really a cause for concern? Do you know why just a cholesterol reading doesn't tell the whole story? Your knowledge about triglyceride, HDL, and LDL may be more limited. What exactly are all these numbers and how do they all fit into the puzzle we've created in this fat-conscious world? Perhaps you'd like to know.

Some of us are genetically destined to premature damage, and others to lead long, energized lives. Either way, nature is determined to get rid of us and make room for younger models. We were designed to grow, mature, procreate, raise our young, and step aside. Our DNA strands carry the necessary information of when to instigate and accelerate our decline. None of us should seriously quarrel with our ultimate destiny, but we at least have the right to try to delay the process a little and enhance the quality of our intervening time.

The propensity for lipid abnormalities is but one among a group of long-term killers that nature inserted into our genetic profiles. When joined by those for hypertension, obesity, insulin intolerance, and diabetes, they form a formidable team of assassins. We've alluded to the metabolic syndrome (Syndrome X) in earlier chapters. This is a significant topic for this book. Combined with the inactivity imposed by fibromyalgia, we face formidable enemies indeed. We want you to recognize them and do something about their ugly intentions.

Arteriosclerosis (hardening of the arteries) is humankind's prime assassin now that antibiotics and vaccines can vanquish most illnesses. It always works with stealth, attacking coronary arteries and causing heart attacks, the number one killer of both men and women. If we escape this fate, similar damage may still wither our brain vessels. This hardening of cerebral vessels is responsible for strokes or can sufficiently impede circulation to cause the serial pinpoint scars that accumulate to produce senility. Also menacing is the circulatory failure that progressively limits locomotion. Kidneys are frequently affected but usher in a slow demise with more warning than the suddenness of cardiac or cerebral shocks.

Arteriosclerosis adversely impacts us by interfering with the blood's delivery systems to the affected tissues. The greatest harm is done as this gradually cuts down on oxygen availability. It also guarantees a rationing of nutrients that can be transported to those areas. Though it's a snail-paced process, all supplies are systematically compromised. Avoiding this late stage requires an early commitment to prevention. Once damage to arteries is fully developed, it's too late to alter significantly. Though coronary arteries can be grafted or cleared, and stints put in to prop them open, nothing can be done to repair the entire system.

We've already led you somewhat superficially through some physiologic concepts. They're far more complicated than our limited discussion suggested. This entire book is filled with our simplifications. While our descriptions may still seem a bit too involved at times, we've attempted to streamline the language to let you better understand the inner workings of your body. Even so, the stepwise chemistry needed to explain minuscule facets of cellular metabolism is often overwhelming. It's no different with the intricacies of fat digestion and postabsorption distribution systems. Let's give it a go anyhow.

It's a commonly accepted misconception that lipid abnormalities are best corrected by following a diet that restricts saturated fats and high-cholesterol foods. Unfortunately, this approach doesn't work very well, simply because only a relatively small part of our circulating cholesterol comes from what we eat. Actually, the liver is the main source of cholesterol in our bodies and the largest internal producer. Quite often, decreasing intake simply goads the liver to replace a perceived deficit by making a little extra. That's sort of the price we pay for the genetic traits that make us each different. People stuck with such metabolic behavior may have to consider the use of medication.

Triglyceride is synonymous with fat and is quite unlike cholesterol, which is a sterol. We bunch them together when we inaccurately speak of lipids, since cholesterol is included. No harm done really, because the problem and the solution remain the same. Low-fat diets are even less help in lowering triglyceride excesses. These, too, arise mainly in the liver after conversion of sugars and starches to fatty acids. It's done as a means of preserving them as a different form of energy. The liver also produces large transport vehicles we refer to as VLDLs (very low-density lipoproteins) that can be used for exporting and ferrying newly formed fats. They're destined for storage mainly in fat cells, and to a lesser extent in other tissues such as muscles. For this reason, abnormal levels of triglyceride are independent risk factors for arteriosclerosis and all of the dire consequences of that condition.

We're going to tackle the problems posed by what we consider bad lipids. We aren't only limited to the above cholesterol and triglyceride. There is a third, deeply involved member: the good guy, HDL. You really need to know some of the habits of this trio to understand cholesterol levels.

CONFUSED? WHAT ARE FATS, REALLY?

> Call it the Big Fat Lie. Fat, has, through no real fault of
> its own, become the great demon of the American dietary
> scene. It is no myth that one third of Americans are over-
> weight. It *is,* however a myth that Americans are over-
> weight due to excessive fat consumption.
>
> —Richard K. Berstein, M.D., *The Diabetes Solution*

Not many Americans would even pause before answering the
question, "What are fats?" We've been bombarded and conditioned on the subject for years. The mere appearance of the
greasy, slimy stuff on our dinner plate evokes an almost knee-
jerk response. Our scrape-it-off attitude was kindled by fire-
and-damnation sermons leveled at us by physicians and the
news media alike. We've been urged to avoid frying, buttering,
or creaming anything we eat. Obediently, we learned to trim
all identifiable fats, and even skin our poultry. We cook using
a few drops of olive oil and do so very sparingly. We dissect
food with forks and knives searching for hidden offenders as
though this activity alone would provide free supplemental
health insurance.

What's so horrible about fat that it strikes such fear in us?
It has certainly been indicted of major offenses against hu-
manity, particularly weight gain and arteriosclerosis. We all
agree that the combined effects of undesirable lipids are the
major cause of heart attacks and strokes. We also pointed out
earlier it's the same circulation problem that causes the premature demise of diabetics. This should qualify fat as a criminal
of the worst kind.

We've been taught to recognize fats and consequently

know they're not easy to avoid. People are well aware that they lurk inside animal products—the very ones that provide us most of our protein. They're also essential inclusions in vegetables. We extract them to get the oils we use for frying and flavoring. We have no method of completely avoiding them. And most of us don't really want to.

We've also been taught that simply eyeballing fats won't tell us what kind they are. We've heard of scary things like transfats and other strange breeds. Only diet savants and nutritionists seem to know what's safe to eat. Laws mandate that food containers be labeled with nutritional contents. Manufacturers flaunt a "low-fat" designation as if it were a medal of honor. They usually succeed in getting us to avoid fattier, competing products by feeding on our fear. The listed fat inclusions glare at us like so many alleged miscreants. These lipid offenders have been posted on so many wanted lists that they're now household words.

Fats are generated from many look-alike fundamental components. They all have a bunch of carbon, oxygen, and hydrogen atoms. How those bits and pieces get strung together is what determines their chemical names. Like our bodies, fats have a spine, but this one isn't bony. It's a product derived from sugars (actually glucose) and is named glycerol. It's like a supporting stanchion for a structure that extends three arms. That's why fats are grouped under the generic name triacylglycerol, something you recognize better as triglyceride. They're simply constructed, with a single glycerol that hooks on three various kinds of fatty acids. Each of these separate appendages has an identifying name. Such attachments can be of different density, length, and weight, and can even be exchanged one for another. Whether they came from animal or plant sources, such attributes are used to determine their various names.

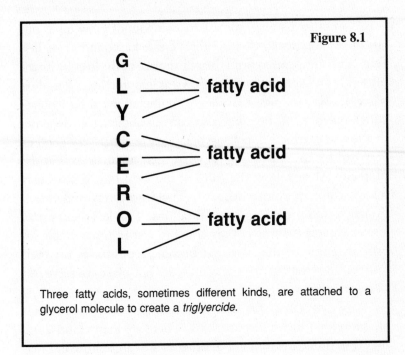

Three fatty acids, sometimes different kinds, are attached to a glycerol molecule to create a *triglyercide*.

Cholesterol, by contrast, is an only child. It has no immediate family members but does claim a few close relatives. None of them is actually a fat, but, as we mentioned earlier, they belong to a group called sterols and steroids. This is an imposing clan that includes many quality members such as the hormones cortisone, estrogen, and testosterone. Other remote kin are also of considerable importance to our bodies, but let's not bring them into this discussion. All are born from the cholesterol molecules that form chemical frameworks for many construction alternatives. Just as we've seen with proteins and fats, hormones are different from each other because of the components tacked onto the basic cholesterol structure.

As in other families, some fatty compounds grow up as pillars of metabolic society, and others create havoc in our bodies. Fatty acids are escorted from their birthplace in the liver by hitching a ride on large fat globules known as lipoproteins. From their name, it's easy to guess that they're combinations of fat (triglyceride) and protein, but they also contain cholesterol. Together they're like chemical double agents. They're either very good or very bad for us, depending on what their inclination is at the moment. Most follow the rules of the road but, disastrously for us, some are more hellbent. These go astray and intentionally avoid programmed destinations. This lets them prowl aimlessly, and eventually they come to rest in unfavorable locations. Some of the sites that become repositories for their fatty cargo—such as arterial walls—are not places to serve our best interests.

As we've stated, the designated functions of lipoproteins are somewhat like transport ships. There are many kinds, and they're as different from one another as are cargo ships and tugboats. They vary greatly in their construction and design. The sturdiest ones have more protein and less fat incorporated into their infrastructures. Their task is to deliver certain goods to preassigned destinations. The optimal vessels for carrying triglycerides are those known as VLDLs. Fat cells provide the safest ports where these transports can be efficiently unloaded. There are usually no delivery problems in the smaller coves offered by various muscles, including the heart. As we've already learned, each of these tissues stores fat as fuel for future energy production.

There's always a little extra fatty cargo below the VLDL decks that is destined for delivery to less active tissues. This is less important for our discussion. What is detrimental for us is when VLDLs get off course and deliver cargo to unscheduled areas that are not prepared to receive it, especially in such quantities. As the name would suggest, the "very low density" of VLDLs describes their lighter weight and even suggests their weaker build. Too often they leak fatty acids onto the wrong destinations, such as arterial walls.

There are also many smaller ships—the LDL class, or the low-density lipoproteins. Cholesterol is the main cargo on these exclusive transports. It's distributed around the body to serve as raw material to be used in construction. Cholesterol will be converted to hormones, or inserted into cellular membranes, or even poured out into the intestines along with bile. Incompetent piloting sometimes endangers an LDL, its crew, passengers, and cargo. When steering goes awry, the chartered vessel has the nasty habit of unloading short of the dock. Left to float the rest of the way, this cargo simply washes ashore onto the walls of the arteries where it remains—and that's not good!

Cholesterol isn't shipped out only on LDLs. It is also loaded by greedy profiteers aboard the VLDL fleet, where it weighs down the ships transporting fatty acid passengers. When this overload is discovered by safety inspectors, it's dumped overboard in order to return the ship to its proper weight. In the haste to dispose of this unwanted cargo, some triglycerides are carelessly shoved off the deck as well.

The Coast Guard may rush forth to protect a few of these cowering survivors and pick up some of the spilled cargo. These rescuers are the HDLs or high-density lipoproteins, and they manage to wrest some of the castaways from danger. Though their vessels are small, they're big enough to take on quite a few of the lighter-weight shipwrecked cholesterols.

These salvaging HDL vessels transport their rescued cargo back home to the liver. There, cholesterol is used, or simply extruded into the bile or destroyed. Unfortunately, the HDL Coast Guard ships are small and can't pick up very much of the abandoned cargo or rescue enough of the fallen passengers.

Shipwrecked triglycerides join cholesterol on arterial walls. Local natives known as mononuclear cells closely protect their territory. They send SOS signals asking for help from assorted fellow villagers. They mount a combined attack and capture the newly beached invaders. The attacking scavengers drag their prisoners into the depths of the arteries and cannibalize them. The intruders can still cause much mischief, however, by causing a biochemical indigestion. Their captors disgorge the fatty remnants into the underbrush, analogous to the inner walls of our arteries. Together, captives and captors alike induce swelling and attract the calcium that eventually hardens arteries and further imperils blood flow. That's how vital organs get progressively deprived of oxygen, nutrients, and, ultimately, energy. This is arteriosclerosis: a hodgepodge of lipids, cellular remnants, and reparative debris that narrow the crucial waterways.

You've now met the entire cast. The assembling of lipids and their transport systems are directed by the body with the best of intentions. Biologic systems are geared for survival and amply endowed to shrug off wild swings in most mineral or chemical insertions. Though we humans are built to last, our genetic predisposition may have set some of us up for premature catastrophes. Others of us simply do ourselves in because of overindulgence. Just as function seriously falters for lack of raw materials, it equally collapses when burdened with oversupply. And thus develops the danger in prolonged association with too many members of the fat family: cholesterol, triglyc-erides, and lipoproteins.

> . . . it begins when its victims are much younger. An oft-quoted study of soldiers killed in [the] Korean War re-vealed that some three-quarters of these young men already had some atherosclerosis in their coronary vessels. Varying degrees of it can be found in virtually every American adult, having begun with adolescence and in-creasing with age. . . . An atherosclerotic artery has been compared to an old length of much-used, poorly main-tained pipe whose diameter is lined with thick, irregular deposits of rust and embedded sediment.
> —Sherwin B. Nuland, *How We Die*

WHERE ARE THE HIDDEN DANGERS IN FATS?

In virtually all the societies in which it is suggested that high fat causes heart disease, the main dietary modifica-tion in this century has been an increase in the con-sumption of sugar, high fructose corn syrup, and white flour—all refined carbohydrates. Surgeon Caption T. L. Cleave who wrote the classic study *The Saccharine Disease* argued convincingly that increases in coronary artery dis-ease could be traced to increases in refined carbohydrate intake. He noted that diabetes, hypertension, ulcers, gall bladder disease, varicose veins, colitis, and heart disease to name a few are all virtually nonexistent in primitive cultures until refined carbohydrates are introduced into the culture. The process took twenty years to develop and so Cleave proposed the Rule of 20 years—that's how

long after sugar or other refined carbohydrates are added
to a culture before diabetes and heart disease begin to appear in that group of people.

—Robert C. Atkins, M.D.,
Dr. Atkins' New Diet Revolution

We'd better continue with our story, since we've only partially
discussed lipid metabolism. Now we know that the body has
systemwide distribution systems and receiving centers. As
we've seen, fatty acids are mainly used for nourishing tissues.
That's why they're launched into the bloodstream. Packaged as
triglycerides, they're sent out for storage and anticipated energy
requirements. Cholesterol is dispatched to places wherever
cells need restoration or remodeling. It's also directed to construction sites located in distant glands such as the adrenals,
ovaries, and testes to be used as raw materials for hormone production.

Returning to our story where we left off, we shouldn't totally condemn the scavenger cells. They initially set out with a
noble purpose, which is to protect and care for their territory.
They begin by snatching some of the stranded fat molecules to
keep them from clogging arterial blood flow. They gobble up
mainly cholesterol, but also a small amount of triglyceride. But
being truly greedy, they even show some appetite for life raft
remnants, the broken bits and pieces of lipoprotein. Whatever
remains after the efforts of the HDL fleet becomes fair game
for these little cannibals. When they become sated and
bloated—as we all do after a full meal—they try to find a place
to rest. The softest spot is directly at hand. They sink blissfully
into the silky-smooth lining of the nearest artery.

The overstuffed scavengers sometimes arrive in droves,

enough to cause bulges in the arterial wall. Not only that, they don't lie still for very long. Frightened at their exposure, they hide by burrowing deep into the arterial wall. The force of their entry squeezes out some of their lipid contents and causes injury to the local environment, because it stimulates fibrous tissue growth that permeates the arterial wall like so many tiny scars. The end result of these scars is that the minuscule muscles in those conduits enlarge as though trying to muster enough strength to squirt blood past points of impending obstruction. These combined changes constrict the waterway and in time greatly narrow the artery.

Disaster sites eventually attract calcium phosphate, as we learned in chapter 2, on fibromyalgia. In the artery walls, it's in crystal form, similar to flakes in the bottom of water kettles or tartar on your dental surfaces. This adds to the clogging and eventually begins closing off the current flowing downstream. As oxygen and nutritive supplies dwindle, cellular function is seriously compromised. Body areas that were once adequately served by these waterways now begin to struggle for existence. This is when we start referring to *hardening of the arteries*—a term that aptly describes the status of these now calcified blood vessels.

IS THERE A SIMPLE SOLUTION?

After ten months on the diet, I had blood work done for my cholesterol. My overall cholesterol had dropped from 221 to 210, but my HDL had increased from 42 to 52. On the diet I eat all the things I avoided for so many years like eggs, sausage, bacon, and cheese. And my numbers got better! The most dramatic change was my triglycerides. Over ten months the number had dropped from 185 to 81. With the weight loss as well my blood pressure started coming down.

—*Cris, Sault Ste. Marie, Michigan*

When asked how to correct cholesterol and lipid abnormalities, most patients will say, "Just stop eating fat." Unfortunately, this is the same answer too many doctors would also give. That knee-jerk statement is only sometimes correct. What seems obvious isn't necessarily true.

Many people can lower plasma cholesterol by sticking with a low-fat diet. Lucky ones might even get a 5 to 15 percent correction. Yet there are lots of patients who would have scant success even if they ate with total dedication to scraping every fatty tidbit off their foods. To make matters worse, a high cholesterol value isn't always abnormal, as we provocatively posited earlier. That's really confusing, isn't it? Let's finally make some sense of this statement.

To accurately decipher what's going on in the bloodstream, what we really need to know is how much of the bad cholesterol is hanging around in the wrong place. The only way to accurately determine this is by finding out how much LDL is in the area. LDL, or low density lipoprotein, is the actual bad molecule that causes the damage. That's the bottom line, and we'll show you how to figure it out.

When reviewing reports on blood lipids, knowledgeable doctors look at more than just the cholesterol value. They know that this one test could be out of what the laboratory flags as normal range and yet be perfectly satisfactory. The reason is that a single cholesterol value is a somewhat misleading number. We also have to know how much protection is available from HDL. Cholesterol measurements detect both good (HDL) and bad (LDL) bunched together as if they were one and the same, and the result is reported as the total cholesterol. Certain lab chemicals are then used to separate out and clearly identify just the HDL component. That provides two distinct values that doctors quickly scrutinize. Then we simply deduct the HDL value from that total cholesterol. We're left with a lesser value that's a step closer to telling us how bad the situation is.

One more obstacle interferes with our pinpoint identification of the threatening LDL. If you recall, the transporter VLDL also carries cholesterol cargo stashed with the triglycerides. Technically we know that, quite consistently, about 20 percent of the load on the VLDL transports is cholesterol. Our last step, then, is to take 20 percent of the VLDL value and deduct that number from the total cholesterol, just as we did with the HDL. Completing this last bit of math gives us an accurate reading of what is truly the bad cholesterol.

Here's how we can state the formula mathematically:

$$LDL = Cholesterol - (\frac{triglyceride}{5} + HDL)$$

This is important, so let's be a bit repetitious and break this down in another way without the analogies. Look at the above formula. To get an accurate reading of the LDL (or bad cholesterol molecule) we need to first complete the calculations inside the parentheses. You'll notice that triglyceride is divided by five. That's because 20 percent of it, or one-fifth, represents hidden but less dangerous cholesterol. Next, add the HDL to the results of that division. Then simply deduct those combined results from the cholesterol, and you end up with the LDL.

Let's do a for-example. Let's say your total cholesterol reading is 210 mg./dl. This reading is flagged as abnormal and you're nervous and you want to see what your actual LDL reading is. So your first number is the 210. Next, you have to perform the mathematical sequence that's inside the parentheses. So you refer back to your lab tests and find your triglyceride reading of 130. You now have to divide this 130 by 5, which leaves 26. Next look up your HDL or good cholesterol. Let's say you're blessed with a nice high 74. Add the 74 and the 26 to get 100. This now is the number that you subtract from the total cholesterol reading of 210. This leaves you with 110, or a normal LDL.

A favorable medical target for this value is below 130. Statistically, there are many fewer heart attacks below that level. Physicians usually urge more stringent efforts for those who've already suffered cardiac misadventures. For them, a value nearer one hundred is desirable. We hope this lets you understand values you're shown after such testing. You should now be able to help in making an intelligent attack on whatever the unraveled abnormalities: LDL, triglyceride, or HDL, alone or in combination.

> More than 2 million Americans have some degree of heart failure that restricts their activities and undermines their vitality. Thirty-five thousand people will die of it annually, far fewer than the 515,000 who will succumb to an actual heart attack, but a large number nevertheless.
> —Sherwin B. Nuland, *How We Die*

Remember also what this book is about, and that's energy. As you've learned, good circulation is imperative for all tissues to receive supplies to rebuild, repair, and be nourished. A heart attack caused by a blocked artery is an extreme. Long before such a crisis, blood vessels all over the body are narrowed and supplies are less than optimal. Arteriosclerosis threatens energy long before it gets as far as threatening lives.

We all know the feeling of a cramp when we try to exercise and we're out of shape. What causes that cramp is the lack of oxygen reaching the tissue. Interestingly, this is the same mechanism that causes a heart attack when an artery is occluded or closed by the calcifications and debris known as plaque. It's on a different scale, but it's really the same scenario in extreme.

We hope we haven't implied that all cholesterol or triglyceride is bad. You certainly need both fuel (triglyceride) and raw material (cholesterol). They're both deeply involved in safe and healthy metabolism. Triglycerides are made available for quick releases of fatty acids to meet energy demands. As we've seen, cholesterol is a basic compound that can be transformed by various chemical attachments to manufacture other molecules and certain hormones. Along with several members of the lipid family, it's also fundamental for maintaining structures. The body works best within normal ranges and sluggishly on either side of those limits. Too little of something is bad; so is too much of anything. That's why doctors focus so much on numerical test results. LDL is just one such meaningful measurement. It helps us keep a close eye on the transport system so necessary to keep energy flowing through our bodies.

Here I am down thirty-five pounds; my blood pressure is 120/80 without medication where it was 140/100 with medication. My cholesterol is down from 220 to 120. My personal doctor had heard of Dr. St. Amand in 1999, and when I asked about going he told me to "save your money." He's now sending *his* patients to Dr. St. Amand.

—*Marty R., California*

Let's get on with the treatment of excessive cholesterol. It often requires a two-pronged approach. Dietary measures avoiding saturated fats (mostly of animal origin) are one method well known to almost everyone. We readily identify meat fat when we see it. For example, it's obvious in the rim surrounding certain cuts of meat, in cold cuts, and in the fatty ripples in a slab of beef. Eliminating such things along with poultry skin, butter, cream, regular milk, and cheese *may* favorably alter the next blood test. A showcase minority of people display dramatic results simply adhering to this discipline. Unfortunately, it's too often not so since the human spectrum is made up of so many genetic variations. Responses to diet alone are quite unpredictable.

Patients who fail on a low-fat diet are usually offered drug control. Humankind was truly blessed with the advent of the "statins." These drugs interfere with the action of a distinct liver enzyme and effectively block production of some cholesterol. They rarely fail to work, and they have few and infrequently seen side effects in the dosages usually required. True, a few people suffer muscle pains or liver disturbances. Physicians are well alerted to these possibilities and usually monitor patients with blood tests, especially in the early phases of treatment. The combination of diet and medication is highly successful and is well documented with saving many lives.

Triglyceride abnormalities should be managed quite differently. They don't respond to the same tricks we use for cholesterol. However, diets are far more successful in correcting triglyceride abnormalities than they are for cholesterol. It's unfortunate that patients are often given bad advice. They're too often simply told to avoid fats and given a corresponding meal plan. This won't work, since much circulating triglyceride is not derived from eating fatty substances.

Let's briefly revisit the mechanism of triglyceride formation even though we've already described the fate of ingested carbohydrates. When the sugar or starch we've just eaten is converted to glucose, the liver scoops it up. It has a good read on what peripheral tissues need at the moment. If there are no incoming signals requesting immediate supplies for outlying districts, the liver determinedly warehouses whatever it can. It's easily saturated, however, with the storage form of glucose, glycogen. Once its own storehouses are well loaded, it still remains keenly intent on energy conservation. Glycogen can't be stored in sufficient quantities anywhere in the body to meet all eventual demands for energy. Much larger power equivalents must be accumulated in more compact form elsewhere.

Wherever sugars are retained, they must be accompanied by significant quantities of water. In fact, if we had to keep even one-quarter of our total energy reserves as carbohydrate, we'd quadruple our weight. Fat doesn't behave that way even though it contains more than double the number of calories. As you already realize, it actually repels water. That makes fat the ideal storage form of energy and fuel reserves. The liver is in full compliance with this body metabolism. When it decodes no messages for glucose export, it rapidly converts excess carbohydrate to fatty acids and expedites them to fat cells as reassembled triglycerides. We've already discussed the packaging and transportation systems that accomplish this.

How many times and for how many years have we been urged to eat complex carbohydrates in lieu of fats? For many people, this was never very sound advice. It was certainly not proper for diabetics, hypoglycemics, and high-triglyceride or overweight individuals. We've already dealt with the "affluenza" now epidemic in the Western world. There is continuing difficulty in grasping the deleterious effects of the highly recommended carbohydrates. The obvious obesity epidemic should prove sufficient, but even this glaring evidence is still being ignored. It shouldn't take a mastermind to decode the problem behind America's expanding girth.

We've fully discussed destructive effects caused by sugars and starches on diabetics. Likewise, we stated that the correction of hypoglycemia was impossible without shunning the more potent carbohydrates. And now here we go again preaching the same doctrine for another health hazard, elevated triglycerides. In genetically predisposed people, eating sugar and complex carbohydrates forces the liver into its energy-conservation mode. You can't get around the biochemical fact that these foods promote the production of triglyceride.

To make matters worse, when triglycerides rise in the bloodstream, the good lipoprotein, HDL, drifts downward. When genetically impaired individuals indulge in carbohydrates, the liver rushes to construct VLDL. Such escorts will be badly needed for transporting the new glucose-to-fat production aimed at the storage containers in fat cells. With these new transporters in place, HDL travels through the bloodstream but doesn't find much loose cholesterol to collect. With no apparent rescue work to do, some HDL sails off to the salvage yard. Not only are the superfluous good lipoproteins destroyed, but the liver perceives a diminished need and stops building them. So you can see how eating too many carbohydrates compounds the problem.

There's an excellent chance that most blood lipids will become normal by your simply avoiding carbohydrates. We know the diet dramatically lowers triglycerides and favorably raises HDL, but it has unpredictable effects on the LDL. If you recall, 20 percent of the VLDL is cholesterol. Some of that percentage will disappear during dieting. Increasing HDL availability helps draw some cholesterol from its dangerous perch on the LDL as well. Those beneficial changes often offset the possibility that eating extra fat allowed in the diet *might* unfavorably impact the LDL.

Even in the presence of high cholesterol, we suggest correcting both the HDL and triglyceride first, since they respond very quickly and visibly within one month of dieting. Then, in a few weeks, simply test the blood and recalculate the LDL. If your individual genetic endowment is such that the LDL remains abnormal, you could still continue the diet and mount a separate attack on cholesterol. Thus, while continuing to slash carbohydrates, you would then also eliminate some of the more obvious saturated fats from your diet. We admit that those dual deletions put tough constraints on anybody's menu. In the long run, we think it far easier to continue avoiding carbohydrates and resolve any remaining problem with anticholesterol medications.

Decisions! Decisions! They must be made, and you have powerful allies to help you. First and foremost, your physician probably understands this biochemistry. You will need medical guidance, but we hope we've primed you enough that you can use your own intelligent approach to change any bad dietary habits. The two of you, allied with accurate laboratory monitoring, are all that's needed to win what should no longer be a simple game of chance. Arteriosclerosis is one energy thief we can't apprehend after the crime. Like the other diseases we've looked at, it's invisible, but it's real. You know enough to believe in things you can't see—just like fibromyalgia. So believe in this one, too, and get started correcting this problem.

OBSTACLES TO OUR SOLUTION

> Let's look at that Frenchman again, the fellow with his teeth buried in the pâté de foie gras. As anyone who's been to France or watches "60 Minutes" knows, the French are far less afflicted by obesity and heart disease than Americans. Yet their diet is *higher* in fat. (They eat comparable amounts of meat and fish, four times as much butter, and twice as much cheese as Americans.) What does it all mean? Could it have anything to do with the fact that the American per capita consumption of sugar is 5½ times that of the French?
>
> —Robert C. Atkins, M.D.,
> *Dr. Atkins' New Diet Revolution*

Low-carbohydrate diets don't often create problems unless you have a serious health issue, such as kidney failure. That's why you always need to check with your own physician just to make sure you're in reasonably good health.

In the context of this chapter, on a low-carbohydrate diet the fact is that your LDL could rise, stay the same, or fall significantly. At the worst, you end up with two improved measurements even if the LDL should go in the wrong direction. Such a trade-off is still preferable to carrying three simultaneous abnormalities, since we can safely treat the abnormal cholesterol sitting on the ever-dangerous LDL. It's also possible that depending on your genetic disposition, your HDL could fail to rise very much even when your triglyceride levels plummet. That, too, might require patients to accept medication. The formula we earlier described sorts out what's good and what's bad. It either provides corroboration for a dietary success or underlines what remains to be addressed.

We've described a *strict* low-carbohydrate diet in chapter 5, on obesity—the diet we prescribe for weight reduction. For some patients, losing body fat might be all it takes to lower cholesterol. Please keep in mind that fat cells and other tissues will release lipids during weight loss. For this reason, testing is often misleading during the correction process. Patient and doctor might wish to delay blood sampling during that reversal time. When you've reached your target weight, that's the time to test your lipids and determine what their real levels are. If you don't need to lose weight, the liberal diet for hypoglycemia is the one for you to use. You can retest about two months after beginning the diet to check your new and improved levels.

We appreciate the catastrophic feeling some people get when they're asked to give up long-cherished goodies. If that's a pitfall to our proposed solution, so be it. We have no way around this, as we discussed in chapters 3 and 5. It's our self-assigned task to offer solutions to metabolic problems; we can hardly be blamed for what causes them.

You've now sifted through a few chapters since we first explored the glitch in energy formation caused by fibromyalgia.

While reading these pages, you must have grown aware of our redundant theme. We've persisted in suggesting the same diet in one chapter after another. It should be clear by now how we feel about health constraints provoked by our carbohydrate excesses. That one tactical, dietary maneuver abolishes hypoglycemia and attacks obesity. It also parries the thrust of insulin resistance and, if timely, banishes the specter of diabetes lurking in its footsteps. Those combined benefits should be sufficient cause for rejoicing and be fully appreciated as formidable successes. They're sweetened in this case by the reduction of dangerous lipid levels, and the resulting lack of damage done to arteries and other blood vessels.

Lastly, as we alluded to above, lowering your intake of carbohydrates may not strip cholesterol off the killer LDL. In that case, it's true that medication might be required. Even so, some type of medical intervention would still have been necessary without the diet. To those averse to taking drugs, we can only reiterate what we said in the beginning of this chapter: Nature is bent on killing us, and has programmed our demise into our genetic code. We in medicine apply whatever skills we possess to *delay* that finality. But more than that, we shouldn't be content with just a long life; we should do our level best to live one free of the debilitating illnesses that sap our energy. It's the difference between being a tired observer and a vibrant participant.

CHAPTER 9

Exercise, Really?
Yes, Really.

In junior high school I had a science teacher named Mr. Ackroyd who was one of those teachers you never forget. He was a dashing former pilot who wore a leather bomber jacket to class, and all the girls had crushes on him. He made us all promise that if he came to us on our deathbeds we would still be able to repeat the basic rules of physics. One of them I remember every time I exercise: "An object at rest tends to remain at rest. An object in motion tends to remain in motion." I have no idea now whose rule that was, but I as I force myself out of the house at the end of the day to do my exercise I repeat it as my mantra. As much as I wish it weren't true on some of those days, I know it is.

—*Claudia M., Los Angeles, California*

If I don't have energy, how am I supposed to exercise?" It may seem that we're trying to beat a dead hen into laying eggs, but we have to insist on another correction. If you were an avid exerciser before fibromyalgia took its toll, then you remember what workouts were like. If you're still exercising, then you can skip this chapter, or read on for a pat on the back. If you're not exercising, then you probably think that any added motion is more than you can bear. It really isn't. In fact, we're going to show you how and why exercise will add to your energy rather than depleting it.

Over the past forty-five years, we've heard many unusual definitions of *exercise.* Raising the issue with patients, we've heard responses such as "I chase my two-year-old around all day," or, "I walk from room to room and constantly go up and down stairs in my house." Gardening with its attendant bending, pulling, and digging is a pastime that's usually given a lot of merit. If you're really doing those things, we'll concede that's sort of exercising. But do those things really result in all the benefits that real prolonged efforts produce?

The truth is that, hard as those efforts may be on the arms and legs, they deliver only marginal cardiovascular or pulmonary benefits. The muscles you're using may get strengthened, but the heart and lungs remain somewhat pedestrian. We'll concede that any activity is better than steady bottom parking in a favorite recliner, but it's hardly the fast lane toward enhanced energy. As you begin to repair your health, it's essential to reenter the world of motion—slowly at first, but with consistency. If possible, go at it with a good attitude. Fix your gaze on certain goals.

Experts divide exercise into two basic categories. One is described as *aerobic*—a word that signifies that oxygen will be needed. We can't ignite a candle without that precious element, and neither can the body long stoke its metabolic furnaces in its absence. You've noticed this for yourself all your life. How far can you dash without needing more oxygen? The opposite word, *anaerobic,* literally means "without oxygen." What this means in terms of exercise is that, unlike aerobic exercise, it is not fueled directly by oxygen. Instead, it's sustained by the energy stores in the muscles, and how much energy is stored there dictates how much you can tolerate.

Most exercise, of course, combines the two forms. During aerobic exercise, there is a point where your oxygen supplies run out, and you start to use your stored fuel from the muscles. On the other hand, at a certain point when you're doing anaerobic exercise such as weight lifting, you'll feel yourself gasping for air. The better shape you're in, the less you'll rely on the muscles' limited amount of stored energy, and the sooner your body will bounce back from any efforts.

As we've stressed earlier, any food can be converted into energy. Sugars are best suited for the quick spurts. Without oxygen, it takes so much ATP (the unit of energy discussed in chapter 1) to break down glucose that we only end up with a small net increase at the end of the process. It's not a very efficient system. It's like driving off on vacation with an eighth of a tank of gasoline. But by tossing a bit of oxygen into the reaction, we can generate thirty-two new ATPs, a much larger net increase. This is like instead taking off with a full tank. That's the difference between anaerobic and aerobic metabolism.

The body stores only a very limited supply of glucose. The liver hoards most of it as glycogen and shares it with other organs as needed. Muscles pack in a little extra as well. The carbohydrate combustion system was designed for very quick and short hauls. It can also handle slower, sustained functions. The body uses an aerobic metabolism day and night for stoking our basal energy fires. The brain is an example of a slow user. On the other hand, strenuous physical effort quickly exhausts reserve glucose tidbits and progressively depends on alternate fuels for energy. That's when fats and a few unused protein remnants have to kick in. Exercise stress also speeds up breathing and sucks in the oxygen required for driving maximal ATP production. And it all happens regardless of which food-derived fuel we end up using.

GET UP AND GET FIT!

Numerous studies have shown that for those who regularly take moderate exercise their life spans are increased. Fortunately, these studies also show that you don't have to exercise very much in order to obtain the benefits.

In other words, moderate physical activity such as regularly walking 30 minutes per day will do you almost as much good as high level activities.

—*www.heartsavers.co.uk*

Despite well-understood links between physical inertia and heart disease, obesity, diabetes, and cancer, America continues to sit. A recent report from the federal Centers for Disease Control and Prevention clearly states the problem. From 1990 to 1998, only 25 percent of adults aged eighteen and older met that agency's criteria for basic physical activity. The standard calls for at least a thirty-minute, moderate-intensity exercise five days a week. This was equated with simply brisk walking, hardly a superathletic endeavor. Alternatively, the agency suggested that more vigorous activities would be equally effective if performed for at least twenty minutes three days a week. Neither undertaking is of marathon proportions, yet most of us blatantly ignore these minimal recommendations.

Some people who now exercise regularly began their routines because of rapid decline in their physical stamina. Others were driven by the sad contour of their bodies. Considerably fewer responded to appeals from their physicians who expressed concern about an obvious deterioration. New Year's resolutions are popular, though not many of them result in a permanent integration of exercise into lives. In truth, all beginners have at least realized they should drive themselves if they expect to regain some well-being. You may be at this early stage and have so far done nothing about it. You know who you are. You're the one always looking for the elevator when the stairs are right in front of you.

We sympathize with the all-too-human seduction of inactivity, but compassion doesn't imply approval. Lifelong habits of sitting and resting are understandably imposed by the fatigue of simply making a living. We each have a long, private excuse list we're happy to share with anyone who asks. The bottom line is that *sedentary* ways are *sedative*. In fact, those two words have the same root derivation. Inertia begets incremental fatigue—the opposite of what you'd expect. Excess rest is like a tranquilizer, whereas exercise actually forces energy into your reluctant system.

We've all been systematically bombarded these last many years by all-too-accurate descriptions of what happens if we don't exercise. If you're like most people, you've probably rationalized such warnings and refuse to give up your seat. However adept you are at holding fast, it's not too late to change.

But there's more. Exercise *isn't* just a means of prolonging life expectancy, although statistically that does seem to be a strong benefit. If it were, it wouldn't be included in this book. This book is about energy, not about extending your life. A long life without vitality gets pretty empty. It takes a heap of strength to satisfy cherished ambitions.

We want to give you more reasons to break through the starting gate and get you going—doing something *active*. Would it surprise you that a brisk walk on a weekend afternoon might at least temporarily erase your mounting sluggishness? Do you know that exercise causes your body to release endorphins, nature's own painkillers? If you're cold, take a walk, and when you come back notice how warm your house seems. Exercise will reset your body's thermostat for you.

WHAT TYPE(S) OF EXERCISE SHOULD YOU CHOOSE?

By far, walking is the form of exercise that people seem most able to easily build into their daily lives without getting bored, and as it provides most of the health benefits for the heart and is well within the physical capacities of the majority of the population it is probably best to adopt it as your main form of exercise if you have no other preferences.

—*www.heartsavers.co.uk/howtoexercise.htm*

As long as you keep moving for at least thirty minutes doing a moderate-intensity exercise five days a week, anything you'll stick to is appropriate for you. An equivalent level would be to do one-hour workouts of your choosing three times a week. Some people feel safest with a repetitive exercise routine. Some get bored too easily doing this and prefer the excitement of variations and tackling something new. It's really up to you as long as you maintain some level of intensity.

There are lots of personal preferences in the exercises we select. It's confusing trying to get started by choosing among the many varieties. Some of us like the slam-bang, let's-go-at-it, I'll-do-it myself approach. Others select the softer but effective touch of yoga, Pilates, tai chi, or the stretch of the passive push-me-pull-you machines that do most of the work. If you don't want to do it alone, there are almost as many places to go as there are exercise variations. You could join classes featured by gyms, studios, community colleges, and local YMCAs or YWCAs.

> I watch a gentle yoga tape and I follow right along with the exercises. When I'm finished, I feel like a million bucks. My mind, my body, and my spirit are just so much better.
>
> —*Eileen R., San Diego, California*

If you're resuming exercise after a long hiatus or simply haven't had much success getting into any routine, consider joining a "returning" or "beginning" class. Remind yourself about doing a few stretches before starting and taking it nice and easy at first. There will be plenty of time later for you to gain momentum and extend the duration of activity. This is meant to be health building, so don't maim yourself right at the starting block. After all those promises to persevere this time and previous false starts, don't beat up on yourself the first day out. You mustn't risk getting discouraged quite so quickly this time around.

Muscles are mixtures of two kinds of fibers: red and white.

White muscle is designed for speed and is primarily anaerobic, so it utilizes little oxygen. It's not the best sort for prolonged effort. Red ones are that color because of their greater blood content and number of ATP-producing mitochondria. They're dedicated to balancing and supporting the body during extended activity. To accomplish this, oxygen is required, and these fibers are therefore aerobic. Since most physical stress uses short or long bursts as well as combinations, different types of fibers are working harder at different times. That's why nature packed mixtures of both red and white fibers, with one type dominant in any given muscle group. It all depends on their intended function. New white or new red fibers can actually develop to match the requirements of chronically resting or heavily exercised muscles.

Obviously, the types of exercise you choose determine what group or kinds of muscles will get the most toning. This choice likewise mainly activates the types of fibers that are doing most of the work and feeds them like a fuel injection system. White fibers like glucose best; red ones will eat anything—sugar, fat, and even protein nibbles. For example, weight lifting is primarily for developing incremental strength and contouring the body beautiful. It uses more red than white fibers, whereas running sprints would develop more white ones. We should therefore design our workouts alternating many different muscles or using most of them simultaneously. Ideally, we should shift gears now and then and give all of the fast- and slow-twitch fibers an equal chance.

Well-planned exercise programs should aim at satisfying three goals. The first priority is to improve and protect the cardiovascular as well as the respiratory systems. Another desire is to promote strength and firm up muscles. Workouts are structured to work against resistance by using repetitive stretching and relaxation. Third and not least is the main thrust of this book: providing a resurgence of energy.

Modern health clubs have multiplied everywhere over the past few years. Most are not terribly expensive. Some are deservedly popular and meet many needs—maybe even yours. These new sweat clubs are well stocked with all kinds of machines and gadgets of various designs. Properly used, they'll make you stronger, develop your endurance, and even nudge your trend toward a morale-promoting shape. Many have enticing swimming pools. They will gladly link you up with classes doing aerobic and anaerobic workouts in or out of the water. Along with other gym members, you may find it much easier going to one place where the routine is tailored for you.

However, you don't really have to join a fancy gym to develop an effective exercise routine. If you're an indoor person, you can simply buy a treadmill and simulate long-distance walking while comfortably reading or watching TV. Of course, if you're an outdoor person, you can just put on a pair of well-broken-in shoes and regularly wander around your own neighborhood. Browbeat or shame some friend into going along if you'd enjoy chitchatting to avoid boredom. It usually strengthens your resolve to use a buddy system.

Lacking such common-interest people, turn to your best friend—the only one that seems happy at the end of a leash. Dogs so quickly develop the walk-and-smell habit, they'll start doing back flips as a gymnastic reminder for getting out of the house. That's a big help when you're tempted to renege on your resolutions.

KEEP DOING IT

> The road back to aerobic exercise is a long and slow one. And at times, it's hard to be patient and start again with ten-minute walks around the block. But it's also a good feeling, even when I'm frustrated. I have my life back.
>
> —*Dorothy McAden, Tucson, Arizona*

However you choose to exercise, stay with your personal goals. Don't let yourself be overly intimidated by career exercisers or bodybuilders. No matter what you've become, you have the power to change it. Only you can do it, and you *can* do it. Make a resolution, and then, as the commercial jargon says, just do it. Don't overthink it, get up and try it. If you get halfway through your walk and it's just too much, then you can stop. But we bet you'll be tempted most days to keep going. Don't make the first mistake, though, which is to stop before you've even started.

TAKE YOUR TIME GETTING STARTED

> Really, exercise isn't very complicated; your body has evolved over millions of years to do regular physical activity, so it's natural.
>
> —*www.heartsavers.co.uk/exerciseforfun*

Luckily, there aren't too many dangers in exercising. Injuries are unfortunately the main ones. It is true that some unexpected twist or turn may seriously stress or even tear a straining tissue. Tendons and ligaments, and less often muscles, are the main victims. You should never become smug or complacent about your mounting skills. Continue taking precautions to avoid any accident that would throw a wrench into your newfound activities. Not only do such disabilities stop your progress, but they also undermine your resolve to resume activities even after recovery. Fibromyalgics often feel that their muscles are more prone to injury because they feel tight, but if you stretch a little, and progress carefully, you should have no special problems.

Professional athletes know better than to leap into activity without some preparation. Stretching before beginning any strenuous activity seems logical enough. This increases the reach of your motor tissues even though it won't totally protect you from injury. When you get to the point at which you propose to run, begin with a progressive fast-walk for a few minutes. That stretches all of the muscles, tendons, and ligaments you will use. Well-done warm-ups will escort you nicely through the physiological, anaerobic limbering-up process that involves the white and red fibers we outlined above. That one to two minutes of muscle flexing is all the time oxygen needs to begin flowing liberally into your system. By then, aerobic energy generation is under way and accumulating at your service.

Regardless of your inherent abilities, instruction and pacing are integral parts of beginning a fitness regimen. Before working with weights or muscle-resistant equipment, ask for an introduction by someone familiar with them. Powerful machines can inflict prodigious stresses and should be treated with respect. The male competitive drive doesn't require much description and is often the novice exerciser's downfall. That guy with the bulging biceps didn't get that way overnight. Make sure you're not trying to lift or pull beyond your current level of prowess. Take it easy. You'll get there in time.

Delayed wear and tear is a common risk for any repetitive sport. Weight lifters face acute dangers of torn ligaments, tendons, and rotator cuffs. These tissues are always susceptible to chronic sprain and spur formation, especially in the neck and back. It's been assumed that joints take excessive beatings from certain exercises. Some studies have suggested that long-term running might induce knee or hip arthritis. Opposing views have appeared in a few medical reviews that found no significant damage even in marathon addicts. Both positions are open to critique. For example, it's possible that injury-prone individuals gave up their marathons before the cutoff date when tabulation began. Others who continued perhaps have inherently better structures.

We won't keep focusing on sports medicine, since there are many better experts on the subject. Our observations stem from our specialty of endocrinology, a field that includes body physiology, chemistry, and metabolism. We're only reporting what we've observed and studied over these past forty-six years, and most of that from being patient-taught. From this vantage level and our own exercise programs, we suggest the following: If during the course of any activity pain begins and is incremental, continuing the effort may lead to damage. Today may not permit the same physical expenditures as yesterday. Women are usually more aware of this than men, because they regularly deal with their monthly, bodily cycles. Men should similarly listen and concede when sophisticated internal and external signals warn of trouble. If any of them strongly suggests *Slow down,* we should be wise enough to listen.

AND THE AWARD GOES TO . . . YOUR BODY!

One day you just have to say to yourself—this is enough, I've felt lousy and I've sat still for too long. And sitting still doesn't make me feel better, in fact, it makes me feel worse because I feel guilty that I'm not taking care of myself. How much worse could I feel if I got up and did a little exercise? I've always said I'm willing to try anything if it will make me feel better, and I just might feel better if I try it. Then get up and try it. Set your sights at something reasonable, and when you meet your goal you'll feel better. Maybe at first you'll feel better just because you're doing something for yourself. And then, keep going. Do it every day, before you have time to think up an excuse. Be kind to yourself if you really feel bad. But try. Like we used to tell the kids, just try it, give it a fair try. Other rewards will come.

—*Steve Stevenson, West Los Angeles, California*

You already know that exercise is the answer—but what's the question? What's the biochemical reward for the body? In brief, what do muscles, brain, bones, heart, and even gut gain by the seemingly abusive behavior we're urging you to undertake? What in the world are we trying to insert into the already beaten psyche of the fibromyalgic?

Simply standing or walking exerts more G forces on the body than allowing chair cushions to absorb most of the stress of gravity. For this reason, nerve and hormonal controls interpret sedentary lifestyles as something akin to partial weightlessness. The less weight bearing is involved, the less the energy mills have to work. Why should the body nudge them into overtime to produce stronger when weaker will do just fine? There's a word for the resulting biologic demolition derby. It's *catabolism,* which means "tissue breakdown." It's the opposite of *anabolism,* which designates "building up of the body."

We undergo subtle changes in posture from age-imposed physical strains, work habits, and just plain living. They're so gradual that we're not aware of the minuscule influence we have on our skeleton from day to day. But the good news is, we're actually able to alter wear-and-tear deterioration to some extent by our behavior. Healthy bones thrive on frequent prodding. Their slow remodeling techniques are simply responses to demands we put on them. Bones adeptly interpret the amount of stress or lack of it that we've selected by our lifestyles. As far as they're concerned, they can grow stronger, weaken and bend a little, or break—your choice. That's why so-called weight-bearing exercise is ordered for patients with osteoporosis, or weakening bones.

A little superficial physiology might help you understand bone games. They harbor some rather large cells called osteoclasts that avidly chew into their ossified surfaces. The jarring of physical stress prompts these cells to begin any necessary realignment. They start the process by taking a few microscopic nibbles, resulting in minuscule defects. They make them just the right size and in exactly the right places according to how they interpret instructions. Multiply those bites several thousandfold over an extended time and you can imagine the potential for bone realignment. All of those tiny gaps must somehow get filled to satisfy any reshaping blueprint.

Different kinds of cells hang around, eager to begin the reconstruction and resurfacing the mini potholes. Osteoblasts, as they're known, carry all the materials and tools of their trade.

They disgorge the correct rebuilding enzymes that layer an undercarpeting of protein matting. Minerals such as calcium, magnesium, sodium, zinc, fluorides, phosphates, and carbonates are then chemically enmeshed and bonded to these surfaces. Added together, they're the bits of new bone we exactly need to repave the deliberately gnawed defects.

Together, osteoclasts and osteoblasts are the yin and yang of bone metabolism. Their destroy-and-repair dance continues throughout life in response to the habitual stress we put on bones. Since exercise more closely mimics the antics of youth, it can even tease aging bones into that rhythmic process. It fools them into thinking young and trying to simulate the growth bonanza of those early years. Studies never fail to show healthy reconfigurations and increased calcium density resulting from punishing bones a bit.

Exercise is like a physiology coach who trains bones into better teamwork with the sinews. The push-pull, yank-and-tug of muscles, tendons, and ligaments is powerfully felt at sites of their skeletal attachments. Worthwhile exercise speaks a metabolic language understood by all osseous structures. Such tissues can't ignore the jarring as long as it's repeated often enough. Bones may not have the finest biochemical hearing, but hammerlike repetition eventually provokes a response. Speeding through workouts may not get the same attention that results from steady and prolonged pounding. Slow but steady more eloquently speaks the demand for beneficial restructuring.

You already know what happens to exercising muscles, and it's no different with bones under assault from weight bearing. The skeleton responds admirably. Bones properly realign and become far better able to withstand demands of simply living.

Exercise sketches an entirely new infrastructure. Newly retrofitted bones are better for support and add to the more aesthetic contour. Along with the rest of our moving parts, a new dynamism develops.

Exercise puts a systemwide and irresistible strain on all companion units—and, needless to say, the response is exceedingly favorable. Exercised sinews, ligaments, and tendons are empowered and strengthened. Together and now more powerful, they exert a greater shearing force upon their bony attachments. As we've just seen, the skeleton has to respond and resist damage by laying down a more resilient mineral glue. We speak of the *musculoskeletal* system with a single word without a hyphen since it defines a unified tissue network. Strengthening a single component of these intertwining structures produces a similarly desirable effect on all cross-connecting supports.

Beautiful muscles and sinews are sufficient rewards for many people, and increased strength only a secondary gain. We must remind you of other progressively relevant gains that also drive the exercise mystique. An accrued sense of well-being provides more than a modicum of that allure. Sooner or later it also dawns on you that you've quite miraculously created a reservoir of energy. It's something new and wonderful that you can tap at will. What's the physiological basis for this bodywide resurrection?

One single muscle fiber may contain as many as one thousand mitochondria, as we discussed in chapter 2, on fibromyalgia. There is now tangible documentation that well-honed athletes may have four or five times more mitochondria in those cells than the couple of hundred found in sedentary folks. When we speak about muscle fibers, we're talking about structures that can only be seen under micro-scopes. Think of the vast numbers included in a total muscle and how many of those there are throughout the body. The more mitochondria we have, the greater our energy reserves. It's now documented that a steady exercise program actually re-builds some of those ATP-making factories.

It may have escaped our attention but we know of few sci-entific data showing improvement of gastrointestinal symp-toms in exercising people. However, those who indulge in even slightly strenuous activity have learned this for themselves. Di-gestion seems better, as does intestinal motility—often suffi-cient to ease or abolish constipation. It's as though gut muscles also enjoy all that bouncing and jostling. These structures also augment their strength of contraction and post gains similar though less obvious than with skeletal muscles. Apparently they, too, can be rejuvenated.

It was recently shown that adult brains, even old ones, are capable of growing new cells. The triggering impetus for this anatomical and intellectual surge came from working puzzles, more complicated math, and written problems. These are surely mental exercises. To our knowledge, no one has yet re-ported that physical exercise would do the same. However, you likely have friends who've succumbed to some join-the-gym promotion and now brag about their restored mental agility. They're usually only too happy to regale anyone who'll listen about their empowerment.

Equally salubrious, particularly for the obese and Type II diabetics, is the biochemical rejuvenation of muscles and fat cells following exercise. You'll recall that resistance to insulin is the earliest manifestation of impending diabetes. Such cellular petulance either diminishes greatly or totally ceases with exercise. Magically, within twenty minutes of working out, muscle cells renew their previously harmonious relationship with insulin. A three-mile walk has such significant impact that this metabolic benefit continues for forty-eight to seventy-two hours. Added to dieting, performing similar drills three times per week would, in the early stages, quite likely avert the impending disaster that is adult-onset diabetes.

RESTARTING YOUR LIFE—THE FINAL PHASE

> Exercise is a miracle drug. Makes you feel better . . . makes you look better. You don't have to be afraid of side effects or interactions with other medications. You don't have to read any package inserts. All you have to do is walk out your door. Walk twenty minutes in any direction and then turn around and go home. And feel proud of yourself. Take some every day, and you'll get better. You can count on it.
>
> —*Gwen M., Santa Monica, California*

If you've spent 90 percent of your life sitting in a chair, walking to the corner Starbucks may seem an admirable achievement. That's especially true when it dawns on you that you must then subject yourself to the return trip. However, you'll probably feel energized for at least an hour or more when you finish. Imagine how pumped up you'd get if you were to sneak up to a full mile, however gradually you achieve that quest. Why not shoot the works? Go for a three-mile stroll and then, over the stretch of a few months, turn that into a fast walk.

Begin the process and see if you, too, succumb to the addictive nature of exercise. It won't be just in your mind! We've only sketchily reviewed what are amazing alterations accruing to the great benefit of muscles, fat cells, bones, sinews, and intestinal and pancreatic beta cells. We've paid scant attention to other structures such as the lungs, heart, and blood-producing elements. Benefits to them from exercise are legendary. It's not news that sexual function is significantly enhanced by exercise. The brain can hardly restrain its profound biochemical exhilaration. It's as though energy had been spliced onto formerly underutilized tissues like little sale tags that pleadingly read USE ME.

Exercise would shape and polish another spoke of your energy wheel. Still, it won't prove sufficient to carry the entire load alone. A detrimental wobble will remain until each spoke is inspected and skillfully repaired. As you'd suspect, precision function demands a smoothly working whole. Exercise is crucial, because its energizing effects stabilize the wheel with sufficient balance for making the other corrections. Replace all defects and your body will reward you with a potent metabolic fix. What's better than perfect health and the vibrant energy to enjoy it?

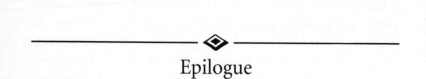

Epilogue

Medical challenges are rewarding and fun for physicians up to a point, and as long as there'll be a happy outcome. Give us a case of bronchitis, a kidney infection, or flu and we're at our best. This is the way we like it: Here's your diagnosis—take this tablet—that's the cure—nice seeing you. No patient skills are involved. Swift results are anticipated, you're happy, and we feel like heroes.

In this book, we've written about a different kind of illness. We, the physicians, *must* have help, and only you can provide it. You'll have to get involved if you plan to change your health. We'll point the way and encourage you when you need it, but that's all we can do. That's what happens when we deal with chronic illnesses. There's no magic pill, no simple solution. You have to be ready to change some things about your life.

Failure to reverse fibromyalgia will leave you exhausted and in continuous pain. If hypoglycemia is ignored, you'll have mood swings, irritable bowel, more fatigue, and panic attacks to add to the mix. And if you don't pay attention to those, you may eventually slip from hypoglycemia into diabetes, aptly named the slow savage killer. Then you'll have no choice but to make radical changes. To add insult to injury, almost all treatments for diabetes result in weight gain. Lipid disturbances will probably appear and require more dietary changes, and more medications. When this happens, it's all too easy to fall for the quick fixes promised by supplements and other expensive potions.

You *can* change the outcome. All it takes is willpower—a heap of it. You'll also need an open-minded physician and a bit of medication. None of these requirements leaps magically out of these pages. *You* must provide the determination and *you* must select the doctor. You may not trust yourself much these days, but somehow you'll have to adhere to a diet and faithfully keep to the prescribed protocol. You'll need to learn to do certain things to take care of yourself. You'll need to make some investments in your own future, like exercising and learning what's best for you.

We began with the analogy of a bicycle wheel. We thought it was a fitting metaphor because of the millions of little energy mills in the cells of our bodies where mitochondrial rotors churn out ATP energy. These power stations must work unimpeded to give us the best energy stores possible within the limitations of our own genetic codes. We cannot be anyone else, but we can be the best it's in our own capacity to be. Wellness is not a competition with anyone else. It's about reaching down inside ourselves and finding out who we were and who we can be again. It's an exciting journey when you're making it in the right direction. We know many patients who think they are better now than they ever were before—patients who think fifty is better than forty, sixty better than fifty, and so on. We carried the wheel reference forward to include the efforts needed for restoration. Fix all of the spokes and, yes, a miracle will just seem to roll into your life.

Resources

◆

CHAPTER 1—MAKING ENERGY

Energy formation and cell biology: vlib.org/science/cell_biology.

CHAPTER 2—FIBROMYALGIA

Books

What Your Doctor May Not *Tell You About Fibromyalgia,* by R. Paul St. Amand, M.D., and Claudia Craig Marek, Warner Books, 1999, has detailed information about the disease as well as the guaifenesin protocol.

What Your Doctor May Not *Tell You About Pediatric Fibromyalgia,* by R. Paul St. Amand, M.D., and Claudia Craig Marek, Warner Books, 2002.

The First Year Fibromyalgia: An Essential Guide for the Newly Diagnosed, by Claudia Craig Marek, Marlowe and Co., 2003.

Fibromyalgia and Chronic Myofascial Pain Syndrome, by Devin Starlanyl, published by Harbinger, is a top seller, both with the old blue cover (1996) and the new, updated green one published in 2001.

Multimedia

A videotape (or video CD) of R. Paul St. Amand, M.D.'s consultation with a new patient, and a demonstration of his mapping technique, is available from The Fibromyalgia Treatment Center, P.O. Box 7223, Santa Monica, CA 90406. All money goes directly into this nonprofit foundation for fibromyalgia research. Tapes are $20 plus $5 shipping and handling.

Web Sites

On-line support group for guaifenesin users: www.fibro myalgiatreatment.com.

United Kingdom On-Line Support Group: uk.groups .yahoo.com/group/UK-FMS-GUAI.

New Zealand/Australia Group: www.vaxau.com/fib.

Guaifenesin Sources

Guaifenesin comes over the counter in 600 and 1200 mg. time-release tablets. At the present time only one company, Adams, is manufacturing it. Other companies' versions may be on the market soon.

There are also 400, 300, and 200 over-the-counter strengths, which are short acting and must be taken three times a day. Updated sources and information will be on www.fibromyalgiatreatment.com.

All forms are available from:

Marina del Rey Pharmacy
Jim Zelenay, Pharmacist
4558 South Admiralty Way
Marina del Rey, CA 90292
(310) 823-5311
e-mail: zelenaymdrrx@aol.com
(The price is approximately $60 for 300 tablets of time-released guaifenesin.)

Immunesupport.com offers the same excellent price for the time-released tablets. Or call (800) 366-6056

Salicylate-Free Products and Information

Personal Basics by Andrea Rose can be ordered from www.andrearose.com, and at (800) 712-ROSE.

Grace salicylate-free toothpastes, mouthwashes, and other dental products. All-natural, tartar-control, whitening toothpastes in several flavors are formulated by Dr. Flora Stay, DDS, author of *The Complete Book of Dental Remedies*, Avery, 1996. Order from www.drstay.com or call (888) 883-4276.

Paula's Choice. Paula Begoun, the Cosmetics Cop, and author of *Don't Go to the Cosmetics Counter Without Me*, Beginning Press, 1996, has a large selection of salicylate-free products on her Web site: www.paulaschoice.com. Or call (800) 831-4088.

Illuminare Cosmetics. Wonderful cosmetics, all with sunscreen and all salicylate-free. Ruthie Molloy, owner. Order from www.illuminarecosmetics.com or call (866) 999-2033.

The Concise Dictionary of Cosmetic Ingredients, 5th Edition, by Ruth Winter, M.S. Crown Books, 1999. See the author's newsletter at www.brainbody.com.

There are lists of salicylate-free products posted at www .fibromyalgiatreatment.com.

CHAPTERS 3, 4, AND 5—HYPOGLYCEMIA AND OBESITY

There are many low-carbohydrate diet resources. Hypoglycemics must proofread all recipes to make sure that they don't contain caffeine or any of the forbidden carbohydrates.

Low-Carbohydrate Diet Resources

Sugar-free products are in abundance on the Internet.

www.lowcarb.ca includes International Yellow Pages and many other resources.

www.lowcarb.com, D'lites of Shadowood, offers low-carb and sugar-free Atkins diet products. Or call (888) 937-5262.

www.86sugar.com offers many products; the flat shipping charge often makes it least expensive.

www.atkinscenter.com, Atkins Nutritionals, Inc. offers Atkins diet products. You can request a catalog by calling (800) 2ATKINS.

www.immuneweb.org/lowcarb offers information for vegetarians.

Low-Carbohydrate Cooking

The low-carb newsgroup is an excellent resource for all low-carbohydrate diets, with links to products, product reviews, and thousands of recipes. www.grossweb.com/asdlc. Now CDs with a recipe book are on sale.

Dr. Atkins' New Diet Revolution, Dr. Atkins' Quick and Easy New Diet Cookbook, and *Dr. Atkins' New Diet Cookbook,* by Robert Atkins, M.D., M. Evans, 2002. The Atkins Center's Web site www.atkinscenter.com has many recipes, seasonal menus, and personal recipe file capacity.

The Low-Carb Cookbook: The Complete Guide to the Healthy Low-Carb Lifestyle with Over 250 Delicious Recipes and *The Complete Guide to Long-Term Low-Carb Dieting,* by Fran McCullough, Hyperion, 1997.

Information about Splenda products is at www.splenda .com or (800) 7-SPLENDA.

Wondercocoa Sugar-free and caffeine-free chocolate for cooking available from www.86sugar.com.

Da Vinci sugar free syrups available from www.davinci gourmet.com. Or call (206) 768-7401 or (800) 640-6779.

Torani Sugar Free Syrups available from www.torani.com and at (800) 775-1925.

CHAPTER 6—DIABETES

For Diabetics or Prediabetics

Dr. Bernstein's Diabetes Solution, by Richard Bernstein, M.D., Little, Brown and Co., 1997. See his Web site at www.diabetes-normalsugars.com.

The First Year Type 2 Diabetes: An Essential Guide for the Newly Diagnosed, by Gretchen Becker, Marlowe and Co., 2001.

Blood Sugar Blues: Overcoming the Hidden Dangers of In-sulin Resistance, by Miryam Erlich Williamson, Walker and Co., 2001.

Rick Mendosa has an excellent, informative Web site: www.mendosa.com/diabetes.

CHAPTER 7—HORMONES

The Anti-Aging Hormones, by Ruth Winter, Crown Publishing, 1997. The author has a newsletter at www.brain body.com.

Woman: An Intimate Geography, by Natalie Angier, Houghton Mifflin, 1999.

CHAPTER 8—LIPIDS

Dr. Atkins' New Diet Revolution, by Robert C. Atkins, M.D., M. Evans, 2002, in paperback has information on cholesterol, lipid, and also blood sugar.

Blood Sugar Blues: Overcoming the Hidden Dangers of In-sulin Resistance, by Miryam Erlich Williamson, Walker and Co., 2001.

An excellent article is "What If It's All Been a Big Fat Lie?" by Gary Taubes, *The New York Times,* July 7, 2002; www.nytimes.com.

CHAPTER 9—EXERCISE

There are abundant resources for you in this category. Basic information can be found at www.webmd.com under Fibromyalgia and Arthritis: Therapy in Motion.

The Arthritis Foundation has three videotapes for sale: *People with Arthritis Can Exercise, Exercise Is the Best Therapy,* and *Fibromyalgia Interval Training* (warm-water exercises). These and various brochures can be ordered via their Web site www.arthritis.org, or by calling (800) 207-8633.

The Oregon Fibromyalgia Foundation has had exercise videos tailored for fibromyalgics for many years. There's a new one (2002) for stretching, in addition to their aerobics video and toning and strengthening video. Sharon Clark, M.D., and her husband, one of the top fibromyalgia researchers, Robert Bennett, M.D., are featured in the new one. www.myalgia.com; (503) 892-8811.

Inside Fibromyalgia, by Mark Pellegrino, M.D., Anadem Publishing, 2001, has information on physical conditioning and some basic exercises.

MORE INFORMATION

Medline: www.medlineplus.gov

Common Natural Salicylates

❖

**To be avoided in topical products and
medicinal preparations
(dietary avoidance is not necessary)**

Acacia
Acerola
Achillea
Acorn
Adder's tongue
Adonis vernalis
Agar
Agave lechuguilla
Agrimony (*Agrimonia*)
Ajaga
Alehoof
Alfalfa
Algae
Algin
Allspice
Almond (oil)
Aloe (vera)
Alpine cranberry
Althea root
Amantilla
Amaranth (*Amaranthus*)
Amber
Ambrette seed

American centaury
American desert herb
American hellebore
American ivy
American mountain ash
American saffron
Amica
Amyris
Anemone
Anethole
Angelica
Angostura bark
Anise (aniseed)
Annedda pychogenol
Apple (blossom)
Apricot
Arbutus extract
Arnica
Aromatic bitters
Arrowroot
Artemisia annua
Artichoke extract
Arum

Asarum
Asclepias
Ash
Asparagus (root)
Aspen
Astragalus
Atlas cedarwood
Avens
Avocado
Babassu
Balm (mint, lemon balm)
Balm of Gilead extract
Balsam (mecca, oregon, peru, tolu, etc.)
Bamboo
Banana
Baneberry
Baptisia
Barberry
Bardane (*Bardana*)
Barley grass
Basil
Bay laurel
Bay leaf
Bayberry
Bean
Bearberry
Bearded darnel
Bear's garlic
Bedstraw
Bee balm extract
Bee pollen
Beech
Beechdrop
Beetroot
Belladonna
Bennet's root
Berberis
Bergamot

Betony
Betula
Bilberry complex/extract
Bilva
Birch
Bird's tongue
Birthroot
Birthwort
Bisabol
Bistort
Bitter almond
Bitter cherry
Bitter orange
Bitterroot
Bitterstick
Bi yan pian
Black alder
Black birch
Black cohosh
Black currant
Black haw (bark)
Black mustard
Black pepper
Black root
Black thistle
Black walnut
Blackberry
Blackwort
Bladder wrack
Blazing star
Blessed thistle
Blind nettle
Bloodroot
Blue cohosh
Blue flag
Blue-green algae
Blue gum eucalyptus
Blue vervain
Blueberry leaves

Bogbean
Bois de rose (oil)
Boldo leaf
Boneset
Borage (oil)
Borneol
Boronia
Boswellia
Bougainvillea
Bourtree
Boxwood
Brahami
Bran
Brassica
Brazilian guarana
Brazilwood
Brier hip
Brigham tea
Broad-leaved peppermint
  eucalyptus
Brooklime
Broom oil
Bryony (*Byronia*)
Buchu
Buckbean
Buckthorn
Buckwheat
Bugle weed
Bugloss (extract)
Burdock (root, extract)
Butchers' broom
Butterbur
Buttercup
Butterfly weed
Butternut (root, bark)
Cabbage (extract)
Cabbage rose
Cabreuva
Cacao

Cactus (*Cactus grandiflorus*)
Cade
Cajeput
Calamintha
Calamus
Calendula
California poppy
Calophyllum (oil)
Camellia (oil)
Camphor
Canada root
Canadian balsam
Canaga
Candleberry
Candlenut tree
Candock
Canenula
Cannabis
Canola oil
Capers
Capsicum
Caraway
Cardemom
Carline thistle
Carnation
Carnauba (wax okay)
Carrot (oil, seed)
Cascara sagrada
Cascarilla bark
Cashew nut (oil)
Cassia
Castor (bean, oil)
Catechu
Catharantus
Catnip
Cat's claw
Catuaba
Cayenne
Ceanothus (extract)

Cedar
Celandine (extract)
Celery (seed)
Centaury (*Centaurea*)
Chamomile (camomile)
Chaparral (extract)
Chaste tree
Cherimoya
Cherry (bark, pit, pit oil)
Chervil
Chestnut
Chia (oil)
Chickory
Chickweed
Chili
Chimaphila
China bark
Chinese angelica (root)
Chinese hibiscus
Chinese magnolia
Chinese tea
Chives
Chrysanthemum
Chuan xin lian
Cilantro
Cinchona
Cinnamon
Cinquefoil
Citronella
Citrus (seed, seed extract)
Clary sage
Cleavers (cleaverwort)
Clematis extract
Clove
Clover
Club moss
Cocoa
Coconut
Cohosh (root)

Cola (nuts, seeds)
Colchicum
Colombo
Coltsfoot
Columbine
Comfrey
Condurango (extract)
Coneflower
Copaiba balsam
Copal
Coral root
Coriander
Corn mint
Cornflower
Cornsilk
Corydalis
Costus
Cottonseed (oil)
Couch grass (root, root extract)
Coumarin
Cowslip
Cramp bark
Cranberry
Crane's bill (extract)
Crataegus
Crocus
Cubeb
Cucumber
Cudweed (extract)
Culver's root
Cumin
Curcumin
Curled dock
Currant
Curry
Cyclamen
Cyperus
Cypress
Daisy

Damask rose
Damiana
Dandelion (leaf, root)
Date
Davana (oil)
Deer tongue
Delphinium
Desert tea
Devil's claw
Dill
Dinkum (oil)
Dock
Dog poison
Dogbane (dogsbane)
Dog's mercury
Easter rose
Echinacea
Elder
Elderflower
Elderberry
Elecampane
Elemi
Eleuthero
Elm bark
Elymus
English ivy
English oak extract
English walnut
Ephedra
Epimedium
Ergot
Erigeron (oil)
Escin
Esculin
Estragon (oil)
Eucalyptus
Euphorbia
Euphrasia (euphrasy)
European ash

European centaury
European vervain
Evening primrose (oil)
Everlasting
Exotic basil
Eyebright
Fava bean
Fennel
Fenugreek (foenugreek) (seed)
Fern
Ferula
Feverfew
Feverweed
Feverwort
Field poppy
Fig
Figwort
Fir needle oil
Flavonoids
Flax (seed, oil)
Flowering spurge
Fo-ti
Foxglove
Frankincense
Fraxinella
French basil
Fringe tree
Fumitory
Galangal
Galbanum
Galega
Galium aparine
Gallweed
Gan mo ling
Garden balsam
Garden spurge
Garden thyme
Garden violet
Gardenia

Garlic
Gay gee
Gentian root
Geraniol
Geranium
German chamomile
Germander
Ginger
Ginkgo biloba
Ginseng
Goat weed
Goat's rue
Goldenrod
Goldenseal
Goldthread
Gotu kola
Gourd
Grape leaf
Grapefruit
Grapeseed
Gravel root
Great burnet
Great periwinkle
Green bean
Green tea
Grindelia
Ground ivy
Groundsel
Guaiacwood
Guar gum
Guarana
Guava
Gum karaya
Gum plant
Hamamelis
Hawaiian white ginger
Hawkweed
Hawthorn (hawthorn berry)
Hay maids

Hayflower
Hazel
Heartsease
Heather
Hedge bindweed
Hedge hyssop
Hedge mustard
Hedge parsley
Helichrysum
Heliotrope
Hellebore
Hemlock spruce
Hemp (hemp agrimony, hemp
    nettle)
Henbane
Henna
Hepatica
Herb Robert
Hesperidin
Hibiscus
Holly
Hollyhock
Holy thistle
Honey
Honeydew melon
Honeysuckle
Hops
Horehound
Horse chestnut
Horse nettle
Horsemint (oil)
Horseradish
Horsetail
Horseweed
Hound's-tongue
Houseleek
Huang qi
Huckleberry (leaf)
Hyacinth

Hybrid safflower
Hydrangea
Hydrocotyl
Hydrophilia
Hypericum
Hyssop
Iceland moss
Immortelle
Impatiens
Imperial masterwort
Indian cress
Indian hemp
Indian poke
Indian turnip
Indigo
Ipecac
Irish moss
Ironweed
Ivy
Jaborandi
Jalap
Jamaica dogwood
Jambul
Japanese turf lily
Jasmine
Java jute
Jesuit's tea
Jewelweed
Jimsonweed
Johnny-jump-up
Jojoba
Jonquil
Judas tree
Jujube
Juniper
Kangaroo paw
Kava kava
Kawa
Khus-khus

Kidney bean
Kidney vetch
Kino
Kiwi
Klamath weed
Knee holy
Knotgrass
Knotted figwort
Knotweed
Ko ken
Kola (kola nut)
Kousso
Krameria
Kudzu root
Kuikui (nut, nut oil)
Labdanum
Labrador tea
Lad's love
Lady's mantle
Lady's slipper
Lady's thistle
Lappa
Larch
Larkspur
Laurelleaf
Lavandin
Lavender
Leek
Lemon
Lemon balm
Lemon verbena
Lemongrass
Lemon-scented eucalyptus
Lentil
Lesquerella
Lettuce
Levant styrax
Lichen
Licorice (licorice root)

Lilac
Liliaceae
Lily (lily of the valley)
Lime
Linaloe
Linalool
Linden
Linseed
Lion's foot
Litsea cubeba
Liverwort
Lobelia
Locust bean
Longleaf pine
Loosestrife, purple
Loquat
Lotus
Lovage
Lungwort
Lupin
Lycii
Lycopodium
Ma hsing chih ke pien
Macadamia
Madder
Magnolia
Mahuang
Maidenhair fern
Maitake mushroom
Mallow
Malva
Mandarin
Mandrake
Mango
Marigold
Marijuana
Marine extracts
Maritime pine extract
Marjoram

Maroc chamomile
Marsh tea
Marshmallow root
Masterwort
Mastic
Mate
Matico
Matricaria
Meadow saffron
Meadowfoam (meadowseed)
Meadowsweet
Meliae seeds
Melilotus
Melissa
Mentha aquatica,
    M. piperita, etc.
Mexican dariana
Mezereon
Milfoil
Milk thistle
Milk-purslane
Milkweed
Milkwort
Millet
Mimosa
Mint (all types)
Mistletoe
Monarda
Monkshood
Moringa
Mormon tea
Mortierella
Moss spores
Mother of thyme
Motherwort
Mountain ash berries
Mountain laurel
Mountain maple
Mouse ear

Mugwort
Muira puama
Mulberry
Mullein leaf
Mushroom
Musk rose
Musk-mallow
Muskmelon
Mustard
Myrcia
Myrrh
Myrtle
Narcissus
Nasturtium
Neem tree
Nenuphar
Nerve root
Nettles
New Jersey tea
Niaouli
Nicotiana
Nightshade
Nutmeg
Oak bark
Oakmoss
Oat flower (oat root, oat straw)
Oleander
Olive (olive oil)
Onion
Opopanax
Orange (orange blossom, orange oil)
Orchid
Oregano (seed, oil)
Oregon grape (root)
Origanum (oil)
Orris
Osha
Oswego tea

Pacific yew
Palm oil (palm kernel oil)
Palmarosa
Panama bark
Pansy
Papaya
Paprika
Paraguay tea
Parsley
Pasque flower
Passiflora or passionflower
Patchouli
Pau d'arco
Papaw
Pea
Peach (peach kernel oil)
Peanut
Pear
Pectin
Pennyroyal
Pennywort
Peony
Pepper (oil, black, red, green)
Peppermint (peppermint oil)
Periwinkle
Persic (oil)
Peru balsam
Peruvian bark
Petitgrain
Pettier
Petty spurge
Peyote
Pichi
Pilewort
Pimenta leaf
Pimpernel
Pine (bark, cone, pycnogenol, needle oil)
Pineapple

Pinkroot
Pinus pulmilio
Piñon pine
Pipsissewa
Pitcher plant
Plantago (seed)
Plantain
Pleurisy (root)
Plum
Podophyllum
Poison hemlock
Pokeroot
Pokeweed
Pollen
Pomegranate
Poplar
Poppy
Pot marigold
Potato
Prickly ash (bark)
Pride of China
Primrose
Primula
Privet
Prosperity
Psoralea
Pueraria
Pukeweed
Pumpkin
Purging cassia
Pycnogenol
Quassia
Queen-of-the-meadow
Queen's delight
Quercus
Quillaja (bark)
Quillay (bark)
Quince (seed)
Quinine

Quinoa (extract)
Radish
Ragged cup
Ragwort
Raisin (seed, oil)
Rapeseed (oil)
Raspberry (juice, leaf)
Rattlesnake plantain
Rauwolfia (extract)
Raw honey
Red clover
Red eyebright
Red pepper
Red pimpernel
Red raspberry leaf
Red root
Red sandalwood
Red sedge
Rehmannia
Reishi mushroom
Restharrow (extract)
Rhatany
Rhodinol
Rhododendron
Rhubarb (root)
Rock-rose
Roman chamomile
Rosa californica
Rosa centifolia
Rosa damascena
Rosa eglanteria
Rosa gallica
Rosa laevigata
Rosa roxburghi
Rose (leaves, extract, oil, hips-
     vitamin C source)
Rose bengal
Rose bulgarian
Rose geranium

Rosemary
Rosewood
Rowan
Royal jelly
Rue
Rutin
Sabal
Safflower (oil)
Saffron crocus
Safrole
Sage
Sagebrush
Salicaria
Sambucus
Sandalwood
Sanicle
Santolina
Sarsaparilla (root)
Sassafras
Savine
Savory
Saw palmetto
Shavegrass
Schinus molle
Schisandra
Scotch broom
Scotch pine
Scullcap
Scurvy grass
Sea holly
Seaweed
Sedge root
Senega snakeroot
Senna
Septfoil
Sesame seed oil
Seven barks
Shanka puspi
Shave grass

Sheep sorrel
Shepherd's purse
Shield fern extract
Shinleaf
Shiitake mushroom
Shunis
Silver fir needle
Silymarin
Skullcap
Skunk cabbage
Slippery elm bark
Snakeroot
Snapdragon
Soapberry extract
Soapwort extract
Solomon's seal
Sorbus extract
Sorrel extract
Southern wood
Spanish broom
Spanish moss
Spanish oregano
Spanish sage
Spearmint
Speedwell
Spike lavender
Spikenard
Spinach (extract)
Spiraea (extract)
Spirulina
Spotted cranebill
Spotted hemlock (root, extract)
Spruce (oil)
Spurge
Squaw vine
Squill
St. Bartholomew's tea
St. Benedict thistle
St.-John's-wort

Star anise
Star grass
Stevia (used as an herbal
    medication, not as a sweetener)
Sticklewort
Stiff gentian
Stillingia
Stoneflower
Stoneroot
Storax
Storksbill
Stramonium
Strawberry
Strawflower
Strophanthus
Strychnos
Sumac
Summer savory
Sundew
Sunflower (seed, oil)
Sweet almond oil
Sweet balm
Sweet bay (oil)
Sweet birch
Sweet cicely
Sweet clover
Sweet fern
Sweet flag
Sweet grass
Sweet gum
Sweet marjoram
Sweet orange
Sweet violet
Swertia
Sycamore maple
Tacamahac
Tagetes
Tall oil
Tamarack

Tamarind
Tangerine (oil)
Tang kuei
Tansy
Taro
Tarragon
Tea
Tea tree
Texas cedarwood
Thistle
Thoroughwort
Thuja
Thunder vine
Thyme
Tiare flower
Tilia
Toad flax
Tobacco
Tolu balsam
Tomato (extract)
Tonka
Tormentil
Trailing arbutus
Tree moss
True lavender
Tuberose
Tulips
Tun-hoof
Turkey corn
Turkey rhubarb
Turkey-red oil
Turmeric
Turnip extract
Turtlebloom
Twin leaf
Ultra primrose
Unicorn root
Uva-ursi
Vacha

Valerian root
Vanilla
Veratrum
Verbena
Veronica
Vervain
Vetiver
Violet
Virginia snakeroot
Virginian cedarwood
Virgin's bower
Viscum
Vitex
Wafer ash
Wahoo
Walnut (extract, leaves, shell oil)
Water avens
Water chestnut
Water eryngo
Water lily
Water pimpernel
Watercress
Watermelon
Wax berry
Wax myrtle
West Indian bay
Wheat germ
White birch
White cedar leaf oil
White ginger
White mustard
White nettle
White oak bark
White pine
White pond lily
White poplar
White sage
White weed
White willow bark

Wild agrimony extract
Wild black cherry
Wild carrot
Wild cherry bark
Wild clover
Wild daisy
Wild ginger
Wild hyssop
Wild indigo root
Wild jalap
Wild marjoram
Wild mint
Wild Oregon grape
Wild sarsaparilla
Wild strawberry
Wild thyme
Wild yam (root)
Willow bark
Willow leaf
Winter savory
Wintergreen
Wisteria
Witch grass
Witch hazel
Woad
Wood betony
Wood sorrel
Woodruff
Wormseed
Wormwood
Woundwort
Yam
Yara yara
Yarrow
Yellow curled dock
Yellow dock root
Yellow gengian
Yellow goatsbeard
Yellow jessamine

Yellow melilot
Yellow parilla
Yellow toadflax
Yerba mate
Yerba santa

Yew
Yin qiao
Ylang ylang
Yohimbe (Yohimbine bark)
Yucca

Index

About the Authors

◆

R. PAUL ST. AMAND, M.D., is a graduate of Tufts University School of Medicine. He has been on the teaching staff at the Los Angeles Harbor/UCLA Hospital, Department of Endocrinology, for almost fifty years. He is currently an assistant clinical professor at the UCLA School of Medicine. Dr. St. Amand discovered guaifenesin's use as a treatment for fibromyalgia, and his work is cited wherever the substance is mentioned.

CLAUDIA CRAIG MAREK, M.A., is a medical assistant tutored, trained, and taught on the job by Dr. St. Amand. She has cowritten medical papers with Dr. St. Amand and has counseled fibromyalgia patients for more than fifteen years.

R. PAUL ST. AMAND, M.D., and CLAUDIA CRAIG MAREK are authors of *What Your Doctor May Not Tell You About Fibromyalgia* and *What Your Doctor May Not Tell You About Pediatric Fibromyalgia*.

HYPERTENSION
The Revolutionary Nutrition and Lifestyle Program to Help
Fight High Blood Pressure

KNEE PAIN AND SURGERY
Learn the Truth About MRIs and Common Misdiagnoses—
and Avoid Unnecessary Surgery

MENOPAUSE
The Breakthrough Book on Natural Hormone Balance

MIGRAINES
The Breakthrough Program That Can Help End Your Pain

OSTEOPOROSIS
Help Prevent—and Even Reverse—the Disease
That Burdens Millions of Women

PARKINSON'S DISEASE
A Holistic Program for Optimal Wellness

PEDIATRIC FIBROMYALGIA
A Safe, New Treatment Plan for Children

PREMENOPAUSE
Balance Your Hormones and Your Life from Thirty to Fifty